Healing Your Body Naturally After Childbirth:

The New Mom's Guide to Navigating the Fourth Trimester

Dr. Jolene Brighten, ND

Edited By:
Bryce Hamrick
Mallory Leone

Mallory's Simple Bone Broth Recipe on page 191 was printed with permission from Mallory Leone

Photo Credit: Natasha Gildea

ISBN-10: 0-9968172-0-4
ISBN-13: 978-0-9968172-0-2

DISCLAIMER

The content of this book is intended for educational purposes only. The medical information in this book is not intended to be used in any way to diagnose, treat, cure, or prevent disease. The information provided and interventions discussed should not be used as a substitute for professional medical advice.

Please consult your licensed health care professional regarding your medical concerns and before making any health related decisions.

The Food and Drug Administration has not evaluated the statements and information provided. The nutritional supplements discussed in this book are not intended to diagnose, treat, cure or prevent disease.

The nutrition, herbal and other treatments discussed in this book should not replace conventional medical treatment.

The information in this book does not represent medical advice. In the event you use any information in this book for yourself or others, the author assumes no responsibility for your actions.

DEDICATION

To my son, Bensen. You teach me more about life then I will ever teach you. Thank you for being the light in my life.

To all the mothers who have come before me and will come after me:

May you always feel the love and support you need on your journey of motherhood.

CONTENTS

"Mother is the name for God in the lips and hearts of little children."

–William Makepeace Thackeray

INTRODUCTION

Childbirth is one of the most incredible athletic events a woman's body will ever experience. From the moment of conception through postpartum, your body makes rapid changes, altering chemically and structurally in ways that no other phenomenon requires. Passing an 8-pound human through a very small space is not without effort.

Most women are hyper-diligent about caring for their bodies during pregnancy. And for good reason! They've been told by their doctors to take all of their supplements, eat right, and get plenty of rest for those 9 months.

But historically, there has not been much focus on what happens to a woman in the postpartum phase. Postpartum women need support and tools that are accessible and realistic to use during this time to heal and recover their bodies.

I was inspired to write this book after the birth of my son. I had prepared myself in many ways, but in this journey of motherhood I have found that you can never be fully prepared. I've had many moments of laughter, joy, tears, and frustration.

I've been so blessed to have helped so many women in my practice step into their role as mother and facilitate their healing journey.

As a mother and a doctor, I hope that this book serves to support you in transforming your mother body, in facilitating your healing, and helping you troubleshoot and treat some of the most common symptoms and conditions that arise after having a baby.

HEALING YOUR BREASTS & BREASTFEEDING SUPPORT

It's incredible that we have the ability to grow a small human and then produce enough food to nourish them during their early life. I really am in awe every time I consider how amazing a woman's body is.

And breastfeeding does more than just nourish your baby. It reinforces the sacred bond between you and your child, encourages your uterus to resume its normal size, releases oxytocin, the love hormone, and can help you lose the extra weight that was essential to your healthy pregnancy.

But while breastfeeding is amazing, many moms struggle with it. Breastfeeding can be painful, difficult, and just plain frustrating. But it doesn't have to be and once you've persevered past the first couple of weeks, it gets a lot easier.

Difficulties with breastfeeding do not reflect negatively on your capabilities as a mother. Rather than allowing frustration and discouragement to build, I encourage you to seek help from a lactation consultant or midwife to help you troubleshoot. We aren't born with an innate understanding of breastfeeding and because so much of our society has discouraged mothers from openly breastfeeding, we don't see it modeled as often as we should.

The World Health Organization recommends exclusive breastfeeding for the first 6 months of life and then continued nursing until 2 years of age. Some women wean at a year, some women breastfeed longer than 2 years and none of it is wrong. You'll discover what works for you and your child. And please remember, your nursing relationship is between you and your baby. Other people will have their opinions, but they are just opinions. They don't decide what is best for your baby—you do!

There will be a lot of changes to your breasts, especially in the first 72 hours after birth. Your milk will come in, your breast will swell and well, you may be uncomfortable. But not to worry! There are natural ways to find relief.

Here are some tips to help you make breastfeeding more successful. If you feel like you need more support, get it! Don't hesitate to ask for help.

Breastfeeding Basics: Tips for Successful Feedings

Get Comfortable. Find a chair that has back support and allows your feet to touch the ground. If your feet don't touch, get a stool to prop your feet on. This will help prevent neck and back tension.

Use a Support Pillow. There are specialty breastfeeding pillows that offer support to baby, but you can use any pillows you choose. This will allow you and your baby some additional comfort.

Tummy-to-Tummy. Hold baby close and ensure both your bellies are making contact the entire time. Baby should be brought to you, not the other way around. This will reduce strain on your body and support a proper latch.

Baby's Alignment. Line baby's ear, shoulder and hip to make feeding and swallowing easier. Baby's head should be tilted back just slightly. A chin-to-chest position makes a proper latch difficult.

Hamburger Hold. Wait, what? Grasp the breast, making your hand into a "C" shape so that the breast goes wide like a hamburger. Yes, there are better names out there I'm sure, but hamburger is always how I held the visualization in my head.

Take Aim. Aim the nipple up towards baby's nose so that when it is inserted it is at the back of baby's mouth, stimulating the palate.

Coax a Wide Open. Sometimes babe will only open part way. Avoid trying to place your nipple in a partially opened mouth—trust me, the pain will make you wish you didn't. Instead, rub your nipple across baby's lip to encourage a wide open.

Chin Down, Tongue Down. Look for this position, once baby's mouth is open wide enough and the tongue has dropped down, insert your nipple and the lower portion of the areola (the dark area around the nipple) into baby's mouth.

Fish Lips. Top lip and bottom lip should fan out like a fish. If not, use your finger to gently open them up a bit more.

Baby's Latch: Baby Has an Important Role Too

Latch is very important for your comfort and baby's success. Your baby's bottom lip should extend beyond the nipple onto the areola, the outer portion of the nipple that is generally darker. The nipple should angle up towards the back of the soft palate to the roof of baby's mouth and all the way to the back. When baby is nursing, make sure that you move the bottom lip to get all the way around the areola.

If you are struggling with latch or you have pain every time your breastfeed, meet with a lactation consultant. Sometimes some one-on-one guidance can make all the difference.

Signs of a Good Latch:

- Tongue is visible when bottom lip is retracted.

- The jaw makes a circular motion, rather than a rapid chin movement.

- Chin touches breast.

- You hear swallowing instead of smacking noises.

- Ears wiggle and cheeks are rounded.

- Nipple does not appear flat when baby is finished.

- Baby shows signs of satisfaction: hands open, falls asleep, falls off breast, and appears relaxed.

Engorgement

" I remember when my milk came in. At first the discomfort had me doubting if I should continue breastfeeding. My breasts were incredibly sore, but I realized my body was responding to my baby's needs and honestly, breastfeeding was the only thing that brought me relief. It didn't take long for us to find our rhythm and when I remember wishing I could just stop breastfeeding. I laugh and am so thankful I didn't. **~Jennifer, mother of one**

Within two to three days after giving birth your body will begin producing breast milk and likely a lot of it. When your milk supply comes in your breast will become engorged. Your body is trying to figure out how to meet baby's demand and its initial response is to bring in a whole lot of milk. This won't last forever—your body will, over time, get the supply and demand ratio down.

In the beginning, you and your baby are establishing a rhythm, which will help your body and brain understand what needs to happen. When baby suckles, the breast is stimulated and signals your brain to release oxytocin. Your body then produces more milk. By feeding on demand (when baby is hungry), your body will get a sense of what is needed.

Natural Remedies to Soothe Your Breasts

Cabbage Leaves. Cabbage leaves have been recommended by Midwives, Naturopathic Doctors, and mothers for ages. Place a cabbage in your refrigerator (best bought before baby arrives) so that it is cool. Peel the outer leaf of the head of cabbage. Place one leaf on the inside of each side of your bra to cover the breast completely. The cool cabbage leaf offers relief by increasing blood flow to the area, reducing inflammation and allowing for easy milk flow.

This is also a great remedy for mastitis and blocked ducts (see page 14).

Wear Comfortable Clothing. Underwire bras or clothes that feel too constricting can make your breasts feel worse. Some women feel better wearing a sports bra or no bra at all in the early days of breastfeeding. Equally uncomfortable is a bra or any clothing that is loose and brushes against the nipples causing chaffing.

Sunlight and Fresh Air. Exposing your nipples to sunlight and fresh air for 20 minutes daily will reduce the growth of microbes and encourage the nipples to heal.

Feed Frequently. Allow baby to feed about every 2-3 hours in the beginning. Be sure to change breasts so that both are drained.

Hydrogel Pads. Easy-to-use cooling pads that soothe sore nipples.

Nipple Creams. Having a mouth on your nipple creates trauma to the skin and exposes your breast to a lot of moisture. This is not only uncomfortable, but can leave you susceptible to infection. Applying barrier creams after every feeding can help soothe and protect your breasts.

First, dry the breast, and then apply calendula or other herbal salve to the nipple. Olive oil-based barrier creams tend to be well tolerated by infants and doesn't make them averse to feeding. Clean the nipple completely before breastfeeding again.

Your skin is an important barrier and first line of defense against microbial infections. If you lose that barrier or it's compromised through the microtrauma occurring from breastfeeding, then you're more susceptible to infection. Applying these barrier creams can help you protect yourself.

Calendula salve, which can easily be made at home or purchased, is excellent for helping heal the skin. Calendula is an antimicrobial herb that promotes tissue healing. It is perfect for sore, dry, cracked nipples and can also be used for diaper rash (bonus!). See my homemade Calendula Salve Recipe on the following page.

Nourishing Calendula Salve

Calendula is a soothing, antimicrobial herb. This salve helps heal dry, cracked or irritated tissue. I have used this salve for postpartum skin issues, as well as my son's diaper rash with great success.

Ingredients:

- 8 ounces of calendula oil (make your own or purchase)
- 1 ounce beeswax
- 1 tablespoon vitamin E oil
- Glass jars 2 to 4 ounces

Directions:

Place herbs oil over a double boiler and gently warm. Slowly add beeswax until it melts. If you'd like a firmer salve, add more Beeswax and less for a softer salve. To test, dip a butter knife into the mixture, remove and allow to cool in the freezer.

Once you've achieved the desired consistency, remove from the heat and add vitamin E oil. Quickly pour into mason jars and allow to cool.

Store in a cool room. This salve will keep for about a year.

Yields 8 ounces of salve.

What if my nipples are cracked and bleeding?

You may be able to heal your nipples naturally using nipple creams. However, if this issue persists it may be a sign of improper latch. It wouldn't hurt to speak with a lactation consultant to see if there are any techniques you could employ to help yourself heal. You should see your healthcare provider if you suspect infection—high fever, chills, body aches, red tissue, and/or foul smelling discharge.

You can continue to breastfeed despite the bleeding. The blood will not hurt baby.

Having a mouth constantly on the breast tissue with all of the moisture that brings can be very aggravating to the skin. If pain lasts more than 1-2 weeks or you're very concerned that something's wrong with your ability to breastfeed or produce milk, definitely meet with your healthcare practitioner.

Natural Remedies for Blocked Ducts

Blocked ducts are simply a backup of milk that can't be expressed. Sometimes it feels like a little Super Ball or maybe like a hard or a firm cord in the breast tissue. Inadequate breast emptying can be common with breast pumps, but may also arise from being rushed, feeling stressed, going too long between feedings, compression on the breast, illness, or baby not feeding efficiently. Or maybe there's no good reason and you've got a blocked duct. Whatever the reason, the remedy is to empty the breast.

If a blocked duct goes untreated, it can lead to mastitis so it is best to act quickly.

With all issues related to breastfeeding, please make sure you are staying hydrated with at least 80 ounces of fluid daily—water, coconut water, electrolyte beverages, mineral water, and decaf tea.

Baby Can Help! Place baby on the affected side with baby's bottom lip aligned with the lump you're feeling (the blocked duct). This will help drain the breast and unplug the duct.

Drain the Breast Often. Nurse every 2 hours, beginning with the affected side. Use a pump when finished to ensure all milk is drained. Pumping may not be necessary if baby drained the breast well. Your baby will drain your breast better than a breast pump so always opt for baby over the pump.

Warm Compress. Apply a warm compress, such as a washcloth heated with warm water, to the breast just prior to breastfeeding.

Massage. While breastfeeding, gently massage from the outer portion of the affected breast towards the nipple. You can also do this while breastfeeding.

Shower Massage. Massage the breast in a warm shower and allowing the heat of the water to run over the breast tissue to relieve pain and discomfort.

Potato Poultice. Grate a cool potato and place directly over the blocked duct. Cover with a cloth and allow it to rest against the breast for at least 20 minutes or until it is warmed. The poultice will soothe the tissue while also increasing circulation and helping to relieve the blocked duct.

Lecithin. The general recommendation is 1200 mg 3-4 times per day when there is a recurrent blocked duct. After 2 weeks without blocked ducts, reduce the dose by 1 cap per week until you are no longer taking it.

Natural Remedies for Mastitis

Mastitis is a condition that should be taken seriously. It may begin feeling like a blocked duct, but then the flu like symptoms begin—pain, fever, chills, and fatigue. The breast will be red, hot, painful, and swollen.

Mastitis most commonly occurs within the first 6 weeks postpartum, but can arise at anytime while nursing.

Mastitis is inflammation of the breast, mostly commonly due to infection that has occurred as a result of engorgement or a blocked duct. Bacteria gain access to the breast, generally through breaks in the skin, and make their way into the duct, feeding on pooled milk.

Risks for developing mastitis include:

- Blocked milk duct
- Engorgement
- Rushed or infrequent feedings
- Nipple cracking
- Pressure on the breast
- Excessive stress
- Illness of mom or baby

There are natural ways to treat mastitis. However, mastitis can quickly progress into an abscess, which is very serious and can result in hospitalization.

If you believe you have mastitis, you need to contact your health care provider, as you may need antibiotics. It is also important to have someone monitoring your symptoms, to ensure you have the right medical care.

Not every case of mastitis requires antibiotics and if you rest and take action early, you may be able to resolve your symptoms. If you do require antibiotics, be sure to take probiotics 2-3 hours following your antibiotic dose to ensure your gut flora isn't compromised.

Drain the Breast Often. Offer the breast to baby every 2 hours, beginning with the affected side. If you feel the breast has not been drained adequately, use a pump following nursing. Your baby will drain your breast better than a breast pump so always opt for baby over the pump.

Baby Can Help! Place baby on the affected side with baby's bottom lip aligned with red, tender area. This will help drain the breast and increase milk flow in the affected duct.

Rest is Essential. Your body requires rest when there is an infection of any kind, mastitis is no exception.

Cabbage Leaves. Place a cabbage in your refrigerator and allow it to cool. Peel the outer leaf of the head of cabbage. Place one leaf on each side of the inside of your bra to cover the breast completely.

Potato Poultice. Grate a cool potato and place directly over the blocked duct. Cover with a cloth and allow it to rest against the breast for at least 20 minutes or until it is warmed.

Castor Oil Massage. Massage castor oil into the breast and armpit (there are many lymph nodes in the armpit) of the affected side. Apply moist heat for 10-15 minutes or take a warm shower and massage the breast. All castor oil MUST be COMPLETELY removed before breastfeeding as it can cause diarrhea if ingested by baby.

Probiotics. Consider eating sauerkraut, kimchi, or other fermented foods, as these provide probiotics and prebiotics, food for good bacteria. Taking a high potency probiotic can help your immune system protect you and is essential if you require antibiotics.

Raw Garlic. Aim for 3-5 cloves daily in divided doses. For example, 1 clove with each meal. Chop the clove into small, easy to swallow pieces and swallow like a pill. The active ingredient, allicin is destroyed with cooking so the garlic must be raw to fight the infection.

Vitamin C. Take 1,000 mg. 3-5 times daily until symptoms subside. Vitamin C can cause loose stools, so reduce the dose if this occurs.

Echinacea purpura Tincture. Echinacea is an herb used to treat infections. Take 1-2 dropper(s) full (or 30-60 drops) every 2-4 hours for the first 24 hours then 3-4 times daily. Take the tincture one additional day after symptoms resolve.

Vitamin D3. It is generally considered safe to take 2,000 IU daily during illness. Having your levels tested will guide you in what level of supplementation is best for you.

Your Vitamin D is Baby's Vitamin D

Adequate vitamin D is important for both your health and baby's. Have your levels checked to know if you require supplementation and definitely get out into the sun as often as possible!

Homeopathic Remedies:

Homeopathy is a type of medicine based on the Law of Similars (like treats like). The description next to the remedies are indications for their use.

- Bryonia 30C: Any movement aggravates. Breast is hard with stitching pains.

- Phytolacca 30C: The breast is hard, lumpy, and painful with baby's latch. Pain can radiate to the armpit or other parts of the body. This is one of the most common remedies.

- Belladonna 30C: The breast is very red, hot, painful, and you may feel a little spacey. High fever generally accompanies.

- Hepar Sulp 30C: Breast is extremely sensitive to touch, better warm, and worse cold. Breast is prone to abscess.

To use Homeopathic remedies: 3-5 pellets 15 minutes away from food every 2-4 hours until symptoms are resolved.

If mastitis gets worse or doesn't improve after 24 hours of natural therapy, seek immediate medical attention.

Antibiotics

If you do need to take antibiotics, which are sometimes necessary at no fault of your own, it's important to take a wide variety of probiotics (multiple strains and high potency) 2 hours after every antibiotic dose. If you experience gas and bloating while doing this, please consult your medical practitioner.

If you develop rash, itchy skin or other symptoms while taking an antibiotic, be sure to contact your prescribing doctor as this may be a sign of an allergy.

Natural Remedies for Thrush

Thrush is a term used to describe yeast overgrowth in the mouth. Yeast, most commonly Candida, is the number one cause of thrush. A warm, moist breast is the perfect environment for promoting yeast growth so you can imagine how easy it is to develop yeast overgrowth on your nipple.

Wash Your Bra and Clothing. Daily washing of your bra, shirt, and breast pads is necessary to keep yeast and bacteria at bay. Dry all clothing thoroughly in the sun or on a high heat setting in the dryer.

Dry and Clean the Breast Between Feedings. If you're applying ointments, make sure that your breast is dry first.

Apple Cider Vinegar Rinse. Mix 2-4 tablespoons of apple cider vinegar with ½ cup of water and wash nipples after each feeding. Dry thoroughly.

Avoid Sugar. Avoid eating foods high in sugar, including refined carbohydrates, which feed yeast.

Apply Calendula Oil. If nipples are cracking, use Calendula oil instead of salve to promote healing and to soothe the tissue.

Swab Baby's Mouth with Probiotics. You can use a pinky's dip worth of an infant powder probiotic before feedings.

Natural Remedies to Boost Breast Milk

There is no reason to think you will have difficulty producing enough breast milk. If you do feel you are struggling with a low milk supply there may be some very simple changes you can make. In some cases, low milk supply can be a sign of a greater problem with your pituitary, thyroid, or other medical issue.

It is not uncommon for women to think they are not producing enough breast milk. More often, your milk supply is just fine, but here are some good gauges to tell if you're making adequate milk and if your baby is receiving it:

- You're changing 4-6 wet diapers per day by the fourth day after birth.

- Your baby is gaining weight after their 1-week check-up.

- Baby's mucus membranes are moist.

- Your breasts are full before and softer after breastfeeding.

- Baby's urine is pale, as opposed to dark.

- Baby is content following feeding.

- There may be milk dribbling out of baby's mouth after feeding.

Drink Plenty of Fluids. Aim for at least 80 ounces of fluids every day—water, soups, broths, and teas. Dehydration can be a culprit in reduced breast milk supply.

Eat Adequate Calories. Eat when you're hungry and ensure you are well nourished (see page 147).

Reduce Stress. Whether it is deep breathing, taking a bath alone, or spending time with your girlfriends, make it a priority. Your milk supply may decline if you are experiencing a lot of stress.

Feel Powerful

Need to drop stress, change your mood, and balance hormones quickly? Use the 1-Minute Power Pose. Stand with your feet wide and your hands on your hips like a famous female super hero. Research has shown that high-power postures decrease cortisol and increase feelings of tolerance for stress, as well as making you feel...well, powerful.

Ashwagandha Tincture. 2 droppers full twice daily. Aswhagandha is an adaptogenic herb that helps lower your stress response and improve sleep.

Drink Galactogogue Tea. Galacotgogues are herbs that encourage the production of breast milk.

Supportive Herbs for Breastfeeding Mothers

" I really struggled with breastfeeding. I thought I would just know what to do. I didn't. I felt ashamed, especially when my baby wasn't gaining enough weight. Fortunately, my midwife encouraged me to meet with a lactation consultant. It completely changed everything—my entire relationship to breastfeeding shifted and I felt confident. I really wish someone had told me before I gave birth that it didn't just 'come naturally' to all moms. It took some time to establish my milk and I had to use formula for a few weeks, but eventually I was able to exclusively breastfeed my son. **~Ashley, mother of one**

Blessed Thistle (Cnicus benedictus). This herb is one of the favorites for establishing and enhancing a healthy milk supply. It also has the added benefit of relieving anxiety and reducing postpartum hemorrhage. If you are experiencing slow digestion, drinking blessed thistle in tea form can also help promote healthy gut transit time.

Dandelion Leaf (Taraxacum officinale). Dandelion leaf is excellent at promoting breast milk production and is nutritive, containing iron and trace minerals. Eating the fresh greens lightly sautéed in ghee or coconut oil is the best way to consume this herb.

    " I tried everything to increase my milk, but nothing worked. After Dr. Brighten asked me to focus on caring for myself and I started herbs for my stress, I began to see an increase in my milk production. I had no idea that stress would keep me from feeding my baby, but it did. What I'd want every mom to know is that addressing your stress can make a huge difference in your milk supply and no one talks about that. **~Denise, mother of two**

Fennel (Trigonella foenum-graecum). Promotes milk production while also encouraging healthy digestion and relieving gas.

Fenugreek (Foeniculum vulgare). One of the go-to herbs for promoting lactation, fenugreek is beneficial when trying to establish your milk supply or for giving it a boost later in the postpartum period.

Goat's Rue (Galegae officinalis). In the same family as fenugreek, goat's rue boosts milk production and supports adrenal glands and digestion. The fresh leaf should be avoided because of toxicity concerns.

Stinging Nettle (Urtica dioica). Nettles are rich in minerals, which are essential in healing. Nettles help restore the blood supply when you have anemia. It also eases muscle aches, leg cramps, and backaches.

Red Raspberry Leaf. This herb tones and nourishes the uterus from pregnancy through postpartum. It is a good source of vitamins and minerals.

Hops (Lupuli strobulus). Hops reduce anxiety and create a calming effect in addition to helping with a quality let down.

Red Clover Blossom. Not only does it create rich breast milk, but it also maintains breast health. Red clover can help reduce anxiety, while also providing minerals.

" I wasn't breastfed as an infant and knew this was something I really wanted. It was painful in the beginning, but it didn't last long. I remember every time my little girl would latch I would feel so at peace and in tune with her. This was a bond that I wish I had shared with my mother and now I was able to share it with my daughter. There is nothing like it! I absolutely loved breastfeeding my daughter.
~Rebecca, mother of one

Mother's Milk Tea Recipes

Nutritive Mother's Milk Tea

Rich with minerals and vitamin C, this tea provides nutrients that support a new mother's body and help to increase milk supply. The chamomile and fennel also relieve abdominal gas and bloating.

- 1 ounce blessed thistle leaves
- 1 ounce red raspberry leaves
- 1 ounce dried nettle leaves
- 1 ounce chamomile flowers
- 1 ounce dandelion leaf
- ¼ ounce fennel seeds
- ½ ounce rose hips

Place all ingredients in a bowl and mix. Store in a mason jar.

To brew a cup of tea: Steep 1 tablespoon of herbs in 1 cup of hot water for 10 minutes, covered.

To brew a large batch: Steep 4 tablespoons of herbs per quart of boiling water for 30 minutes.

Drink 1-4 cups daily.

You can enjoy with a small amount honey too!

Calming Mother's Milk Tea

I find this tea to be really lovely before a nap or at bedtime to help relax the mind and body. The combination of catnip, chamomile, lemon balm and lavender calm the nerves and offer a sweet little cup of bliss.

- 1 ounce blessed thistle leaves

- 1 ounce fenugreek

- 1 ounce red raspberry leaves

- 1 ounce catnip

- 1 ounce chamomile flowers

- 1 ounce lemon balm

- ⅛ ounce lavender flowers

Place all ingredients in a bowl and mix. Store in a mason jar.

To brew a cup of tea: Steep 1 tablespoon of herbs in 1 cup of hot water for 10 minutes, covered.

To brew a large batch: Steep 4 tablespoons of herbs per quart of boiling water for 30 minutes.

Drink 1-4 cups daily. If you want to enjoy a relaxing tea without increasing breast milk, leave out the blessed thistle and fenugreek. Fenugreek can be a little overpowering for some women to drink as a tea. You can always take fenugreek capsules instead if this is true for you.

Restorative Mother's Milk Tea

Licorice and ashwagandha help the body rebalance and support glands, such as the thyroid. Milky oats are considered a nervine, which is another way of saying it nourishes and calms the nervous system. The herbs in this tea blend support a healthy mood, energy, and stamina.

- 1 ounce alfalfa leaf
- 1 ounce nettle leaf
- 1 ounce milky oats
- 1 ounce red raspberry leaf
- ½ ounce ashwagandha
- ½ ounce licorice root

Place all ingredients in a bowl and mix. Store in a mason jar.

To brew a cup of tea: Steep 1 tablespoon of herbs in 1 cup of hot water for 10 minutes, covered.

To brew a large batch: Steep 4 tablespoons of herbs per quart of boiling water for 30 minutes.

Drink 1-4 cups daily.

If you have high blood pressure, omit the licorice.

HEALING YOUR VAGINA NATURALLY

During pregnancy many women experience swelling, discharge, varicosities (veins popping out), and other symptoms that affect the vagina. Your vagina is sore, swollen, and in serious need of some TLC. Following vaginal birth, pain, swelling, bleeding, and overall discomfort is par for the course.

The time it will take for your vaginal tissue to heal and recover is variable depending on the extent of the trauma—including if you had a tear or episiotomy. Caring for your body using natural remedies will not only help you recover more quickly, but will also decrease the amount of discomfort you are experiencing.

Early Vaginal Bleeding

Lochia is the medical term for the vaginal bleeding that occurs postpartum. It is normal and you will often see many clots, which can vary in size.

The bleeding generally transitions from red to brown and eventually becomes a yellow or clear discharge. For many women, the discharge will be gone by 4 weeks postpartum, but some may have discharge up to 8 weeks.

If you experience new onset of heavy bleeding or large clots after the discharge has stopped or feel concerned about the discharge, be sure to speak with your healthcare provider.

Do not use a tampon, menstrual cup or insert anything into the vagina during your first 6 weeks postpartum. Instead, opt for organic pads and change often to avoid vaginal irritation.

Natural Remedies to Heal and Soothe Sore Tissue

Sitz Baths. Traditional sitz baths, which consist of having one tub with cold water and another with warm that you alternate between, are the most ideal, but you may not have easy access to a bathtub or even have the energy to set up a sitz bath. Because of this, I recommend a modified postpartum sitz bath utilizing herbs to encourage tissue healing and soothe the area.

Postpartum Sitz Bath. Place the herbs directly into a muslin bag and immerse the bag in the hot water of the bath. To do this, run the bath water with only hot water, place the muslin bag and one cup of Epsom salt into the bath water and allow to steep. Once the water has reached a comfortable temperature you can get into the bathtub. Remember, you only need enough to cover the genital area, so if you're not up for a full bath, just place a small amount of water in the bathtub.

Herbs for Sitz Baths

- Calendula flower: antimicrobial, soothing, anti-inflammatory

- Rosemary leaves: antimicrobial

- Comfrey leaves: promotes tissue healing

- Lavender flower: antimicrobial, relaxing

- Thyme leaves: antimicrobial

- Uva ursi berry: antimicrobial

- Shepherd's purse leaf: hemostatic (stops blood flow)

- Yarrow: antibacterial, antifungal, hemostatic

Choose ½ cup each of four to six of these herbs and place in a large bowl to mix well. Place the herbs in a large Mason jar and store in a cool dry place. When ready to use, take ¼ cup of the mixture and place in a muslin bag for your bath or use any of the following methods.

It's important that you do not apply too much heat or stay immersed in hot water for too long as it can create pelvic stagnation. Consider ending the bath after 20 minutes of heat or when the water cools.

To increase circulation and promote healing, end the bath with a cold compress placed directly on the genital area for 10 minutes or run cool water over the vaginal tissue for 30 seconds.

Making a Topical Tea. Bring two quarts of water to a boil. Add one cup of herbs and remove from the heat. Cover and allow to sit for 20 minutes. Strain and allow to cool. Use as a rinse at the end of your shower.

Note: The herbal mixture will keep at room temperature for about 6-8 hours, in the fridge for three days. *Do not take internally.*

Herbal Peri Bottle Rinse. Place cooled Topical Tea (see above) in a peri bottle. To use, apply a stream of fluid from the peri bottle to the vaginal tissue during urination and following using the restroom.

Herbal Cold Compresses. Apply the Topical Tea to organic pads or reusable organic cloth and place in the freezer. Apply these cold packs to the vaginal tissue, either allowing them to warm or removing after 10-15 minutes. Take care not to over-apply cold compresses.

Apply as often as you find necessary for the first three to seven days.

What if I'm birthing in a hospital?

You can make individual muslin herb bags prior to delivery and store them in plastic bags or storage containers to keep in your hospital bag. In a pinch, you can place them in a basin of very hot water and use both the water and muslin herb bag to cleanse the area once the water has reached a comfortable temperature.

When to talk to your healthcare provider:

If you've had a major tear, trauma, or an infection, please discuss these therapies with your doctor. They may be contraindicated in early postpartum. Signs of infection include fever, chills, nausea, vomiting, extreme redness, tenderness, foul odor, or pus.

Healing Vaginal Tears & Episiotomy

If you've experienced severe tearing, ask your doctor about using a topical antimicrobial following bowel movements and urination. Sometimes, a simple water and iodine solution will be recommended if you don't have an iodine allergy

Keeping a clean peri bottle next to the sink to be used when you void will help decrease discomfort. Fill the peri bottle with warm water and express the water onto the urethra during urination to help dilute the urine to make the sensitive tissue more comfortable.

You can also use the herbal sitz baths wash solution in the peri bottle.

Using the same principles and techniques to heal the vaginal tissue as previously discussed will also improve the healing of tears. Some women have residual pain and discomfort even after the tissue has healed. If this is the case for you, you should consider speaking with your doctor and a pelvic floor physical therapist.

In my practice, I've helped many women to resolve scar tissue and restore their tissue integrity, as well as create more uniform tone.

Healing Vulvovaginal Varicosities (Dilated Veins)

During pregnancy there is a great deal of pressure on the pelvis and, as a result, circulation isn't at its best. Many women experience mild dilations of the veins in the vulvar area. It is not uncommon for these to resolve after pregnancy; however, if they become enlarged, hot, or painful after birth please speak with your doctor.

Sitz Baths. Sitz baths using comfrey, yellow dock, plantain and yarrow reduce swelling and relieve discomfort.

Hydrotherapy. Alternating hot and cold hydrotherapy heals the tissue and increases circulation. For new moms, I recommend performing hydrotherapy in the shower. At the end of your shower, turn the water to cool-cold and apply directly to your pelvis and the affected area. If you have a removable shower head, apply the cold water directly to the veins.

Apply warm water for 1 minute followed by cold water for 30 seconds. Repeat for a total of 3 rounds, always ending with cold.

Vitamin E. 400 IU daily, taken internally to promote antioxidant activity and healing of the blood vessels may be used. You may also apply the oil topically to the affected tissue to soothe and aid in healing.

Bioflavonoids. 1,000 mg daily supports blood vessel integrity to prevent the vein from enlarging further.

Homeopathic Calc Fluor cell salt 6x. 3-5 tabs 3 times daily to stabilize connective tissue.

“ Why don't people tell you how crazy things can get down there? I remember being so swollen and having no idea what to do after I had my baby. The nurse offered ice packs, but no one really talked to me about what more I could do or what had happened to my body. **~Tammy, mother of one**

Preventing Pelvic Organ Prolapse

I recommend that women rest in bed and lay down as often as possible for at least 2 weeks following childbirth. Relaxin, the hormone that allowed your cervix to soften and your hips to widen, can remain in your system up to 6 months after delivery. This is why some women experience joint instability and can be injured with early intense exercise.

Why is it important to minimize time on your feet?

In the beginning, when relaxin is still high, the uterus is heavy, and the pelvic floor muscles are in need of recovery, you are at risk for developing a vaginal and uterine prolapse. The combination of all these factors, plus gravity and the potential overextending yourself can put you at even greater risk.

Refrain from being overly active is the main message I want you to walk away with. Yes, you can grab a snack, use the restroom and engage in very light activity, but in those early weeks really focus on resting as often as possible.

In Chinese medicine they recommend that the feet don't touch the floor for the first 40 days following childbirth. This is a beautiful illustration of the kind of support you'll need in those first weeks after childbirth. Obviously, this is ideal but not always possible.

If you don't have a lot of support and you feel that you need to be on your feet and taking care of things, try taking frequent breaks. Some of my patients have found it helpful to set a timer so that they aren't standing for longer than 20 minutes at a time.

If you feel heaviness begin to develop in your pelvis, take this as a sign that it is time to rest. Sensations of pressure and bulging are common with pelvic prolapse.

Types of Prolapse:

Cystocele (Anterior Vaginal Wall Prolapse): Herniation of the anterior wall (bellybutton side) of the vagina, with or without dropping of bladder.

Common Symptoms: Urinary incontinence or difficulty with urination.

Rectocele (Posterior Vaginal Wall Prolapse): Herniation of the posterior wall (back side) of the vagina, with or without dropping of rectum.

Common Symptoms: Constipation, fecal incontinence, urgency.

Eneterocele: Intestines protrude through or to the vaginal wall.

Common Symptoms: Pelvic fullness, pelvic pain, bulge sensation in the vagina, pain with intercourse, pulling sensation in pelvis that is better with lying down.

Apical Compartment Prolapse: Descent of the uterus or upper portion of the vagina to the opening of the vagina.

Common Symptoms: Urinary incontinence or difficulty with urination, bulge sensation in vagina.

Because the vagina is a continuous organ, it can be difficult to differentiate a prolapse and often there can be an issue with several aspects of the vagina.

Working with a skilled pelvic floor provider to rehabilitate stretched muscles and support the organs of the pelvis will enable your body to heal. Further medical intervention may be necessary and your health care provider can assist you in ensuring your have the necessary care to heal your body.

In my experience, women with pelvic organ prolapse benefit greatly from Holistic Pelvic Care™ and Mayan Abdominal Massage. Uterine prolapse can be quite challenging for many women to resolve, which is why I recommend vaginal massage with Mayan Abdominal Massage.

Holistic Pelvic Care™ is an internal vaginal massage technique combined with mind-body breath work to heal the pelvic floor physically and energetically. This powerful therapy was developed by Tami Lynn Kent, a women's health physical therapist and author of *Wild Feminine*.

While many doctors will prescribe Kegel exercises as a first line therapy in the treatment of pelvic floor dysfunction and prolapse, I urge you to seek help from a pelvic floor specialist. While exercises to strengthen the pelvic floor are a very important part of healing, they are often not enough and when done improperly (which may be due to imbalance of other muscle groups) they can lead to further dysfunction. Meet with someone who will take a holistic approach your pelvis and will evaluate your entire musculoskeletal system, not just your pelvis.

Vaginal Wind

Vaginal wind or the release of air from the vagina is very common in the early postpartum healing. There's a lot of laxity in the tissue. You passed a human through a very small space—which has weakened your vaginal tone. While it can feel embarrassing, it's nothing to be ashamed of. It's very common. Most women experience it.

Performing pelvic exercises can help you regain tone. You may also consider working with a trained pelvic floor professional to increase your vaginal tone.

Because many women feel embarrassed when there is a release of air from the vagina, you may want to practice exercises or yoga moves at home before you go to a class. For example, audible vaginal gas can be passed when moving from down dog (a yoga pose) into another position, and although completely normal it is far from ideal.

Exercise for the Pelvic Floor (aka vagina rehab)

Traditionally prescribed for urinary incontinence, Kegel exercises are only part of the equation when it comes to rehabbing the vagina. Now, I don't think Kegels are bad, but it is important to note that they are only part of your recovery and do have the potential to make symptoms worse when over done, done incorrectly or other issues are present. But engaging these muscles does have the benefit of increasing circulation to the pelvis. Increased blood flow and lymphatic (immune system) flow promotes healing while helping your body fight microbes that could cause infection. Performing gentle Kegels early in postpartum can also help you maintain muscle tone and reduce the risk of other complications, such as incontinence or organ prolapse.

But there are a lot of complications that can arise after a small human passes through the vaginal canal—pelvic pain, scar tissue, pain with intercourse, incontinence, vaginal prolapse. I think you get the picture. And many of these symptoms can interfere with day-to-day life and subsequent pregnancies.

Kegels that are performed correctly can enable your body to heal. I see plenty of women who really have no idea how to do a Kegel. And why would you? It is nothing like a bicep curl. Kegels can be especially difficult to master after you've given birth because the tissues have been stretched, bruised, and are now swollen—a good time to consider getting help from a professional.

How To Perform a Kegel

The first step in performing a Kegel exercise is to identify the target muscles. There are couple approaches to helping you to identify these muscles. I recommend using the one that makes the most sense to you, but you can certainly try both.

Stopping the Flow of Urine. While urinating, stop the flow midstream by engaging your pelvic floor muscles. This is not the actual exercise, but will help you identify the muscles you want to engage. I recommend only trying this once, maybe twice to avoid increasing the risk of a bladder infection.

Examine Your Vaginal Floor. Insert one lubricated finger into the vagina. Contract the pelvic floor so that you feel the walls of your vagina squeezing inward and upward around your finger.

When you're ready, contract the pelvic floor and imagine your are lifting the vagina towards the crown of the head and hold for at least 2 seconds. Relax the pelvic floor completely and then repeat.

Four Common Kegel Mistakes

Contracting the Wrong Muscles. When performing a Kegel, the glutes, thighs and abdominal muscles should be relaxed. The focus should be on the pelvic floor.

Pushing Down Instead of Pulling Up. Bearing down, similar to when having a bowel movement, is a common mistake when performing a Kegel. It may be helpful to insert one finger vaginally so you can feel the direction of the contraction.

Forgetting to Release the Contraction. Relaxing completely is as important as the exercise itself. Maintaining the contraction without relaxing can cause the muscles to become over worked and creates too much tension in the muscles, which may lead to pelvic floor dysfunction.

Lack of Consistency. Like all muscles in the body, consistency is necessary for building strength. Don't give up too early!

Sample Exercise for Pelvic Floor:

1. Contract the pelvic floor, lifting the muscles up.

2. Hold for 2-3 seconds.

3. Relax for 2-3 seconds.

4. Repeat for a set of 5-10.

Start slow and take care not to fatigue the muscles. If you are experiencing urinary incontinence, overworking the muscles can make symptoms worse. It is better to start with a few repetitions and build up to more over time. Listen to what your body needs and be gentle in not overdoing the exercise.

What if I'm having trouble engaging my pelvic floor?

Having an experienced practitioner perform myofascial work (soft tissue therapy) with you as an active participant can help alleviate trigger points and allow you to have a more uniform contraction of the muscles. They can also assist you in learning how to properly engage the pelvic floor in day-to-day life.

Not all pelvic floor issues can be solved with Kegels alone. I recommend working with a qualified practitioner to fine tune muscle imbalances and ensure you do not over strengthen the pelvic floor (yes, that happens) in relation to other muscle groups.

I generally recommend women begin pelvic floor therapy after they've been cleared at their 6-week postpartum check-up. Working with an experienced physical therapist or Holistic Pelvic Care™ provider can ensure your pelvic floor gets the attention it needs and long-term complications, such as pelvic pain, can be prevented.

Is a 6-week Check-up Necessary?

You should absolutely have your 6-week checkup with your doctor or midwife following delivery. This is where they check how the tissue is repairing and healing, making sure that there are no signs of infection and that your uterus is healing properly. It's more than just getting a clearance for sex and exercise. While it's important to know whether your body is ready for these activities, it's also important to have other symptoms evaluated at that time.

Labs to Consider Testing Postpartum

Depending on what your birth was like, your current symptoms, healthy history and family history your doctor may want to order labs anywhere from 6 weeks to 3 months postpartum.

Lab	Evaluation
Complete Blood Count (CBC)	Evaluates white blood cells, red blood cells, and screen for anemia.
Ferritin	Evaluates iron stores.
Comprehensive Metabolic Panel (CMP)	Evaluates liver, kidney, and gallbladder function.
Thyroid Panel (TSH, Total T3, Total T4, Free T3, Free T4, Reverse T3)	Evaluates thyroid function and health.
Thyroid Antibodies (Anti-TPO, Anti-Thyroglobulin)	Screens for autoimmune postpartum thyroiditis.
Vitamin D	Determine vitamin D status and evaluate if supplementation is warranted.
B12 and Methylmalonic Acid	Evaluates vitamin B12 status.
Folate	Evaluates folate status.
Homocysteine	Indirect marker of inflammation that also gives insight into B vitamin utilization.

Lab	Evaluation
MTHFR Gene	Evaluate if there are underlying genetic issues that may affect mental health, energy utilization and detox pathways.
HgA1C	Marker of blood sugar over a 3-month period. Important if you had gestational diabetes.
CRP and/or ESR	Measurement of inflammation
Salivary Cortisol	Determines function and health of adrenal glands.

Natural Relief for After Birth Pains

After birth pains are normal and they can be pretty extreme for some women. They are the result of your uterus contracting back to its original size, a process known as involution.

These contractions generally begin about 12 hours following delivery and may be as mild as your menstrual cramps or as intense as labor contractions. Each time you nurse in the early days following birth you will also feel these contractions. That is because baby's nursing stimulates the release of oxytocin, often called the "cuddle hormone," which causes contractions and helps return your uterus to its original size, among other things. Another benefit to breastfeeding!

In addition to returning your uterus to its original size, these contractions also prevent excess bleeding, which is why it is important to avoid aspirin. Aspirin thins the blood and can lead to increased bleeding.

If you feel like you need to take something for these contractions, try to avoid acetaminophen or ibuprofen as these have side effects that can impact your health, such as leading to intestinal irritation. Instead keep the following remedies near you when you breastfeed to alleviate pain:

Homeopathic Mag Phos 6C. Take 3-5 pellets every 15 minutes for pain. You may find it helpful to take a dose just before you begin nursing.

Hot Water Bottle. Apply heat for up to 20 minutes to the low abdomen. Wrap the outside of the hot water bottle with a towel and avoid making contact with baby.

Cramp Bark (Viburnum opulus) Tincture. Take 2 droppers full just before you nurse. It reduces pain without inhibiting the uterus from shrinking.

Motherwort (Leonurus cardiac) Tincture. Take 2 droppers full up to 4 times daily. Motherwort is a uterine tonic and also eases anxiety, irritability, and supports a healthy heart.

Uterine Massage. Before each time you stand up for the first 3-6 weeks postpartum, massage your uterus. Make your hand into a fist and knead the lower belly. This is a technique that may help decrease the amount of bleeding and help the uterus heal.

Natural Remedies to Heal Urinary Tract Infections

Urgency, frequency, or pain with urination may be a sign of a urinary tract infection (UTI). It is wise to contact your doctor if you experience these symptoms, especially if you have a fever, nausea, back ache, or see blood in your urine. If caught early you may not require an antibiotic. However, if there is any risk of the infection affecting your kidneys you want to act quickly and meet with your doctor, as an antibiotic will be necessary to resolve the infection and protect your kidneys.

Prevention:

- Wear white cotton underwear changed daily

- Use only mild, natural detergents on clothing

- Use non-deodorized, preferably organic, sanitary pads

- Wipe front to back after bowel movement

- Avoid bubble baths

- Shower after swimming

- Avoid tight pants

- Eat lacto-fermented foods 3 times weekly

Natural Treatment of Urinary Tract Infection

Diet: Avoid sugar, alcohol, caffeine, aspartame, and dried fruits until symptoms resolve.

Increase Water Intake: Drink a glass of filtered water every 20 minutes for 2 hours then every hour for 24 hours, except during sleep.

Vitamin C: 1,000 mg 4-5 times daily for two days. Can cause loose stools, so decrease the dose if this occurs. After two days, reduce dose to 500 mg 4-5 times daily for five days.

Cranberry Juice: Drink 4 ounces of unsweetened cranberry juice 4 times daily for 1 week.

Cranberry D-Mannose: 2 capsules twice daily for 1 week.

Homeopathic Remedies:

- Cantharis 30C: Use when there is painful burning with urination.

- Equisetum 30C: Use when there is pain and a sensation that the bladder is always full, despite having just urinated.

- Sarsaparilla 30C: Pain at the end of urination, may not be able to void unless done so standing up.

- Berberis 30C: Painful bladder, relieved by urination.

- Staphysagria 30C: UTI comes on after intercourse.

To use Homeopathic remedies: 3-5 pellets 15-minutes away from food every 2-4 hours until symptoms are resolved.

Urinary Incontinence

You sneeze, you pee. You cough, you pee. You pick up your baby ... and you pee. It is not only inconvenient, but also embarrassing. And it's also a common symptom following childbirth.

Some women will easily recover and will not experience long-term issues with urinations, while others will go on to experience a daily incontinence or urinary leakage.

Kegels (see page 47) are one way in which you can strengthen the pelvic floor to reduce or eliminate urinary incontinence. You may also want to consider meeting with a Holistic Pelvic Care™ practitioner or a pelvic floor physical therapist to help you understanding the muscle imbalances that are contributing to your symptoms (Hint: Kegels aren't always enough.)

If you are having trouble with urine leakage, try bending forward at your waist next time you need to cough or sneeze. This will decrease the amount of downward pressure on the pelvic floor.

Natural Healing After a C-Section

I think it is important to acknowledge that there is no shame in having a C-section. Many women, especially those who were planning a natural birth, feel ashamed and sometimes defeated after a C-section, as if they did something wrong because they didn't delivery their baby vaginally. There is no shame in doing whatever it took to bring your baby into this world and to ensure their health and yours, no matter the procedure.

Regardless of the type of delivery, you are a mother and you have a beautiful baby to be grateful for. You're amazing—today and every day.

For most women, a small layer of skin begins to heal over the wound within 48 hours, protecting it from bacterial infections. However, this skin is fragile and easily disrupted. Typically, women are able to shower after the first 48 hours following delivery.

Please contact your health care provider immediately if you experience pain at the site, fever, discharge from the wound, the tissue becomes red or there is an odor present.

Many women find the following tips helpful in healing from a C-Section.

Keep the wound dry and clean. After your showers, gently pat the wound area dry. Avoid clothing, which rubs against the wound site.

Bone Broth. Drink at least one cup daily. Along with being easy to digest, bone broth is rich in minerals and amino acids to aid your body in healing. See recipe on page 191.

Grass-fed Gelatin. Consume 2-4 tablespoons daily. Another source of amino acids to support connective tissue healing.

Rest and Sleep. You are recovering from a surgery. Take it slow and allow your body time to heal.

Ask for Help. Get help wherever you can to reduce the need to be up and about.

Anything you can get help with to reduce your need to be up and about will allow your body the much-needed time it needs to rest.

" I think a lot of my depression came from feeling so ashamed from having a C-Section. It wasn't what I wanted and I felt like I had done a really bad job as a mother. I definitely felt like a failure. I remember when I first talked to Dr. Brighten about this and her response and encouragement really helped me shift the way I had been viewing my birth. She encouraged me to work with a mind-body therapist to process the event, which really helped. From talking to other moms, I learned that what I felt was really common. When I look back, I'm not ashamed of my C-section— my choice was to have a surgery or lose my baby and possibly my life. It took me a long time to feel confident to say that I made the right choice, but now I really know that I did. **~Alex, mother of three**

Healing Herbal Wash

This herbal wash is antimicrobial, which prevents infections and keeps the area clean. The comfrey and calendula promote rapid tissue healing and healthy skin.

- 2 ounces comfrey leaves
- 2 ounces calendula flowers
- 2 tablespoons Oregon grape root
- 1 ounce lavender flowers
- 1 tablespoon sea salt

Mix the herbs together in a large bowl. Bring 1 gallon (4 quarts) of water to a boil in a large pot. Turn off heat and add 1 large handful of herbs to the pot and stir. Cover the mixture for overnight, strain the herbs and store the liquid in the fridge. It will keep for 3 days.

When you're ready to use, place sea salt in a peri bottle and fill the bottle with the herbal liquid. Shake well.

In the shower, use the herbal wash to gently cleanse the wound area.

You can use this herbal wash daily. In my house, I keep calendula flowers and Oregon grape root on hand to make a quick wound care wash for when my little one gets a scrape.

SEX, LIBIDO AND INTIMACY

If you're reading this shortly after giving birth you may be thinking there is no way you will ever want to have sex again or give birth again. It's hard to think about intercourse when your tissue is swollen, tender, and…well, currently does not remotely resemble the pre-delivery version.

    " What libido? Between the night feedings, exhaustion and trying to adapt to having a baby, being intimate with my husband was the last thing on my mind. It was about 3 months after having my son that my husband asked me if I was still interested in him. Of course I was! I just felt overwhelmed. Once we scheduled dedicated time to be together and I began to feel more support from him, my libido and even my mood increased.
    ~Allison, mother of one

Where's My Mojo?

If you're struggling with libido, you're not alone. Many women are not interested in sex following birth, which has a lot to do with your hormones.

After birth, your estrogen and progesterone levels drop, decreasing your sex drive and even inhibiting your ability to orgasm. In addition, prolactin rises with breastfeeding, further diminishing your sexual desire. This may sound bad, but in fact, it is exactly what your body should be doing. Think of it as a natural birth control.

Speaking of birth control, you can become fertile early in your postpartum recovery. I've had plenty of women in my practice who have become pregnant right away. Because their period hadn't returned, they thought it was impossible. Your period follows ovulation, which means it is entirely possible for you to become pregnant without knowing you're fertile. And breastfeeding doesn't protect you from a subsequent pregnancy, sorry.

In addition to the hormonal changes you're experiencing, you're tired. Fatigue can crush your sex drive. Throw a little stress into the mix and your libido doesn't stand a chance. Working on decreasing stress and getting more rest can be just what you need to revive your sex drive.

Share with your partner ways that they can help you. Most partners don't fully grasp that doing the dishes, tending to the kids, or showing you support can do wonders for boosting desire and creating a deeper connection between the two of you. As women, we need more than physical stimulation, we need to feel loved, supported and appreciated.

If you feel your low libido stems from deeper-seated issues between you and your partner, seek support through a couple's therapist and communicate what you are feeling to your partner. Raising a child is demanding and exhausting for all couples and many couples struggle to find their groove and make the time for true connection.

When There's Pain with Intercourse

Stretching of the perineum (the area between the vagina and anus) alone can leave the tissue sore and tender, especially with intercourse. Add to this the trauma of tearing and possible sutures and you're bound to feel tenderness for weeks or months after birth.

Your pelvic muscles may also feel tender and sore deeper in the vagina due to the stretching and pressure created by birth. Internal vaginal massage and Holistic Pelvic Care™ can help you rebuild and repair these muscles.

Sex can also be a wonderful massage for the muscles. Gentle intercourse can help you connect to your pelvic floor, increase circulation and rehab your libido. But go slowly. There is no need to rush. Take this time to communicate your needs to your partner. Many women are apprehensive to have sex following childbirth, so slow and gentle is a universal desire as you ease your way back into this physical, mental, and emotional experience.

If pain persists, please seek medical care and don't delay on receiving help from a qualified practitioner. With early intervention, many of your pelvic discomforts and physical apprehension around sex can be resolved.

Explore the New Terrain

Your body has changed in some ways and the sensations you experience are different from what you were once accustomed to. Exploring your body to understand what brings you pleasure will help you not only revive your libido, but communicate to your partner what your needs are.

You can also involve your partner in this exploration by trying new and exciting things. Exciting doesn't necessarily translate to "adventurous" activites or moving outside your comfort zone. Maybe there is a place you've always wanted to go on a date. Reading erotic stories to each other, incorporating adult toys or kissing like when you first started dating are examples of ways in which you can get creative with your intimate life. You may be surprised by what you find interesting now that you didn't before.

Be gentle with yourself and please do not put too much pressure on the sexual aspect of your relationship. While it has been my observation that women who are physically intimate with their partners seem to have higher tolerance to stress and a more relaxed demeanor (which may also be the reason they are more physically intimate), it doesn't mean that you can't have some of your needs met through cuddling, hugging, kissing, holding hands, or other means of showing affection. Just be sure to check in that you are indeed having your needs met.

Tips for Partners:

Go Slow & Be Patient. The tissues take time to heal and her hormones can take time to rebalance. Be gentle with her heart and her body.

Don't Take it Personally. If she doesn't seem "into you" it may be more about what she is experiencing then the way you're flirting.

Communicate. Both inside and outside the bedroom— ask her what she needs, likes, desires and share yours too.

Show Your Love with Support. Vacuuming, doing dishes, taking a turn with baby— these are the new sexy. For women, this IS foreplay.

Tell Her She's Beautiful. A lot of women struggle with accepting their "new body" and don't necessarily feel beautiful. Let her know she is.

Reminisce. Recounting to her all the reasons you fell in love with her can stir up some powerful emotions.

Get Help. Being a parent is hard and takes a toll on your relationship. If you're struggling, looking for outside support may be the answer.

Vaginal Dryness

Once vaginal bleeding has slowed, the vagina can become very dry due to changes in your hormones. Intercourse should not be attempted until you've had your 6-week examination; however, if you need relief, try applying vitamin E oil or calendula salve to the vaginal tissue as needed. Even coconut oil can do the trick for some women.

You can begin to have sex after your health care practitioner has examined you and communicates that you have healed. It may take a little longer to get back to sex if you had a substantial tear or other trauma. Be patient with yourself. It is important that you heal.

Oils can be soothing to the vaginal tissue, but should not be used as a lubricant with condoms because they will reduce their effectiveness. Instead, try using an organic personal lubricant that is compatible with condoms. And please remember, ovulation always comes before menstruation. Just because you haven't had a period doesn't mean you are not fertile.

HEALING YOUR DIGESTION NATURALLY

The first bowel movement following the birth of your baby can be intimidating because of the trauma that your tissue sustained during birth. There's a lot of tissue swelling, the area is really uncomfortable, and there may have been tearing or even stitches.

It's almost tempting to try to hold it until the area feels better, but believe me, you do not want to start down the road of constipation. The longer your stool remains in your colon the more opportunity your body has to resorb the water in the stool, making it very hard and difficult to pass.

Hard stools that require straining can cause you to develop hemorrhoids or aggravate them if they are already present.

It is normal not to have a bowel movement during the first 24-48 hours after delivery, but going much longer than that is not recommended. If you find you are unable to have a bowel movement, please contact your doctor or midwife, especially if you had a C-section.

Drinking plenty of fluids and eating soft, easy to digest foods such as soups can help your digestive system adapt to the changes that have taken place following delivery.

Sometimes doctors will prescribe docusate, a stool softener, to help make this first stool more comfortable. If you prefer to go more of a natural route, try some of the following tips.

Natural Remedies for Constipation

Stay Hydrated. Your demands for fluids are much higher while breastfeeding. Be sure to drink plenty of fluids.

Prune Chia Seed Pudding

Eat this as a morning meal or snack on the days your bowels are being a bit stubborn.

- 4-6 prunes
- 1 cup of water
- 2 tablespoons chia seeds
- ¼ teaspoon cinnamon
- ¼ teaspoon nutmeg

Place prunes and water in a saucepan. Cover and simmer for 15 minutes. Allow to cool and place in a food processor or blender with chia seeds and spices. Puree to your preferred consistency. Enjoy warm or cold.

Magnesium. You can take 150-400 mg of magnesium to help soften the stool. The side effect of too much magnesium is loose stools. Be careful not to over do it. Taking too much magnesium can cause diarrhea.

Do not use harsh laxatives. Avoid the use of castor oil or purging buckthorn as both of these are very stimulating to the bowels and can make you very uncomfortable.

Natural Remedies for Hemorrhoids

Many women develop hemorrhoids during pregnancy, either from pushing during labor or from the extensive hours spent sitting while breastfeeding. Yup, most ladies get them, so if you are dealing with them—you are not alone. But that doesn't mean there isn't anything you can do about it!

There are many natural therapies to reduce pain and shrink the hemorrhoid itself.

What are hemorrhoids?

Hemorrhoids are a swollen group of veins or a single vein located in the anal region.

Include Fiber in Your Diet. Eat plenty of vegetables and include 1-2 servings of fruits in your diet daily to help maintain healthy digestion.

Eat Berries. Include ½-1 cup of strawberries, blueberries, raspberries, or blackberries in your diet daily if you're struggling with hemorrhoids. They provide nutrients like bioflavonoids to help strengthen your blood vessels.

Avoid Aggressively Bearing Down. Increased pressure can cause the hemorrhoids to enlarge and become more painful. You want to get the stool to a state where you can sit down and relax and have an easy bowel movement.

Stay Hydrated. Your demands for fluids are much higher while breastfeeding. Be sure to drink plenty of fluids. It is especially important to ensure you are taking in enough fluids if you are increasing your fiber.

Fresh Ground Flaxseed. Combine 1-2 tablespoons into food, smoothies or water daily. They are a source of omega-3 fatty acids as well as soluble and insoluble fiber. Be sure to buy the whole flaxseed and grind yourself in a coffee or spice grinder as pre-ground flaxseed loses its nutritional value quickly. Freshly ground flaxseed can be stored in the fridge or freezer for up to a week.

Witch Hazel Tincture. Apply witch hazel to the hemorrhoid several times daily using a cotton ball. There are many over-the-counter products for hemorrhoids that contain witch hazel and are quite effective at reducing hemorrhoid symptoms.

Prune Chia Seed Pudding. See page 184.

Soothing Sitz Bath

Used externally, yarrow has the ability to stop bleeding and provides comfort with pelvic pain.

- ¼ cup of yarrow
- ¼ cup of calendula
- ⅛ cup plantain

Simmer herbs in a medium size pot for 20 minutes. Strain and pour into a shallow bath. Submerge the pelvis for 15-20 minutes once daily.

HEALING YOUR MOOD NATURALLY

Many women experience anxiety and/or depression following birth. Sometimes the anxiety stems from the fears that come with being a new mom. I've been there too—"Am I doing this right? Am I doing this wrong?"

It's all new and it is perfectly normal to feel anxious about some of the decisions you have to make. I recommend talking with a few people you trust or choosing a couple good resources that you can consult.

The moment you become pregnant there are people lining up to give you advice. While their intentions are well meaning, it doesn't mean that you need to heed their advice or even entertain it. If you feel overwhelmed, excuse yourself or politely let them know, "Hey, thanks, but I've got this." Because you do!

And please, back away from "Dr. Google." The advice I've seen offered to new moms out there is downright scary. I can remember being a couple weeks postpartum and thinking that if I wasn't a doctor and didn't know better then I'd be completely freaking out by what people said.

But sometimes anxiety and feelings of low mood persist. Sometimes your mood symptoms feel debilitating. And sometimes, you need more help than a good friend or family member. It's important to recognize when this is the case. There is no shame in anxiety or depression.

Getting help early on is the biggest gift you can give to yourself and your family. You're not failing. You're not a "bad mother." You're a strong, capable woman who is doing her best and who needs support. We all need support in one way or another. And any mother who tells you it was never hard or that she loved every minute is either not aware of her struggles or is misremembering. And yes, I understand that statement may be upsetting, but the reality is—being a mother is HARD. There are days where it is simultaneously the most wonderful and awful thing I've ever done. I don't regret one moment of it, but it ain't easy.

Postpartum Thyroid Dysfunction and Mood

I recommend all women have their thyroid tested if they are experiencing postpartum depression. Depression is a common symptom of low thyroid hormone.

And other times, your mood is a physiological sign of something deeper. Low thyroid hormone, anemia, inflammation, and adrenal exhaustion are some causes of anxiety and depression in new mothers. Detecting some of these issues is as simple as a blood or saliva test. And catching them early will help you restore your health and prevent other issues from arising.

I recommend working with a Naturopathic Doctor, Functional Medicine Doctor, or Holistic Psychiatrist to understand and treat the root cause. There are many resources available for new moms, including support groups. See Resources on page 211.

Baby Blues vs. Postpartum Depression

Within a few days of birth, an estimated 80% of women experience what is termed "baby blues." Baby blues is characterized by a mildly low mood that lasts about 2 weeks. This state generally stems from fluctuations in hormones and changes to your life as a whole.

Postpartum depression is a more severe form of baby blues and occurs in about 20% of new mothers. It is important to see your healthcare professional if you experience the following symptoms:

- Anxiety
- Chronic exhaustion
- Diminished appetite
- Depression
- Despair
- Difficulty concentrating
- Frequently crying or inability to cry
- Guilt
- Hopelessness
- Insomnia
- Memory loss
- Mood swings
- Panic attacks
- Thoughts of hurting the baby or yourself

Natural Mood Boosting Practices

- Make time to go out and meet with friends.

- Take a light walk.

- Expose yourself to sunlight. If it is winter, purchase a natural light to sit in front of during daylight hours.

- Sleep in a completely dark room.

- Listen to music you enjoy.

- Watch a favorite television show or movie.

- Practice deep breathing exercises, meditation, yoga, and cross body action exercises.

- Try acupuncture, massage, chiropractic, and other bodywork.

- Receive craniosacral therapy.

Feeling Restless? Try Passionflower

Passionflower helps activate GABA receptors in the brain, which can help you feel relaxed, calm and less anxious.

- Meet with a counselor.

- Get involved in a new hobby.

- Laugh often.

- Journal your thoughts.

- Say no and don't feel bad. Set your boundaries and know your limits. Your priority is to heal.

- Journal your thoughts and feelings.

- Rest, not just sleep, but also rest your body.

- Maintain blood sugar balance by eating when hungry and having fat and protein with your meals.

- Try baby wearing to engage in activities while keeping your little one close.

- Dance, sing, and find your groove!

- Get out into nature.

- Hug. Your partner, children, loved ones. Hugs increase oxytocin.

- If you have a pet, cuddle & play with them. (If you don't have a pet, now is not the time to get one.)

- Foster relationships that build you up and ditch those that bring you down.

- Play.

- Blowing bubbles can be highly therapeutic and allows you to interact with older children without having to be too physically active in the beginning. Those deep breaths to create a bubble stimulate the rest and digest aspect of the nervous system. Watching bubbles float and children play can also feel uplifting.

" I really thought I could be super mom. I thought I would need no help and I'd be able to do it all myself. I refused help from friends and would catch up on housework while my baby napped. Eventually I became depressed and felt so resentful towards my husband. I really struggled. It was a hard lesson to learn, but if I could share anything with new moms it would be to get help as often as possible and not to ignore yourself.

~Donna, mother of two

Mood Balancing Nutrition

- Eat protein and fat with every meal.

- Avoid skipping meals.

- Incorporate fermented foods into your diet—kefir, sauerkraut, fermented vegetables, kombucha, and beet kvass.

- Eat four to six eggs yolks per week.

- Consume coconut oil, grass-fed organic butter and other healthy fats daily.

- Eat fatty fish like salmon, mackerel, sardines and anchovies three times weekly.

- Drink ½ cup or more of bone broth daily or combine it into meals.

- Eat offal, especially liver, 3 to 4 times weekly.

- Drink turmeric ginger tea. See recipe on page 164.

- Feed your gut with fiber—fruits and vegetables are a great source!

Digestion is important too! If you are experiencing digestive symptoms—gas, bloating, constipation, diarrhea, heartburn, or any other discomforts in your gut—please meet with a qualified healthcare professional. Skin rashes, acne, joint pain and allergies can also be signs your gut is unhappy. Your brain health is dependent on your gut health. Sometimes the key to improving your mood is through your gut.

" I had to sleep. I just had to. It didn't work for me to be up all hours of the night. I learned that lesson with my first son. When I had my second son I hired a postpartum doula to help me at night. It made all the difference in the world! I had a bit of sadness, but nothing like my first son. **~Chloe, mother of two**

Natural Remedies to Support a Healthy Mind

" My postpartum depression was really bad when I had my son. I didn't want to tell anyone and tried to hide it. I eventually began counseling, which helped, but I think exercise was probably the best thing for me. You spend a lot of time inside with your baby. I think getting outside and exercising really helped me. What I'd want to share with moms is that you shouldn't have to hide how you feel. If you feel bad, talk to someone about that. Depression is really hard, but it is especially hard when you are doing it alone.

~Stephanie, mother of one

Magnesium. 150-400 mg at bedtime supports neurotransmitters, is relaxing, anti-inflammatory, and necessary for adrenal health.

N-Acetyl Cysteine (NAC). 600-1800 mg taken with food. NAC is a powerful antioxidant that supports neurotransmitter health while also creating a more anti-inflammatory environment.

Omega-3 Fatty Acids. Docosahexaenoic acid (DHA) is particularly good for brain health. It is an omega-3 fatty acid found in the brain and other tissues in the body. It plays an important role in activating the growth of new brain cells and is an anti-inflammatory nutrient.

Curcumin. Curcumin is the active ingredient in turmeric. It reduces inflammation, which benefits your mood, your brain function, your digestion and can alleviate muscle aches and pains. It has been used traditionally to enhance breast milk supply. Enjoy in meals such as curry or as a tea. See the turmeric ginger tea recipe on page 164.

Probiotics. There have been multiple studies showing that the bacteria in your gut influence your mood, both positively and negatively. Aim to incorporate probiotic-rich foods, as well as ample fruits and vegetables, which your good gut bacteria love.

Vitamin D. Vitamin D is synthesized by your body when you are exposed to sunlight. However, depending on your current status, supplementation may be necessary. Vitamin D regulates enzymes involved with neurotransmitter production and protects the brain against free radicals. A simple blood test can you help you determine if you require supplementation.

" I felt like I was losing my mind. It started with anxiety and feeling like I couldn't even handle the smallest decision. Several months later the depression set in and I was struggling to get out of bed. My milk supply dropped and my doctor was telling me I needed anti-depressants. I sought Dr. Brighten's help because I didn't want to take drugs for the rest of my life. After ordering labs I was diagnosed with hypothyroidism and needed a medication. At first I was hesitant to begin the thyroid pill, but after 3 days I felt like myself again and my milk supply slowly returned. Dr. Brighten helped me work on what was causing the autoimmunity and I was able to eventually come off the thyroid medicine. I don't know what I would have done had I not found Dr. Brighten.

~Taylor, mother of 3

Herbal Mood Support

" My depression didn't go away until almost 3 years after having my daughter and that is because that is when I finally got help. I went to my Naturopathic Doctor and we created a plan that I was comfortable with. Looking back, I wish I had reached out much sooner.

~Jill, mother of one

Gentle Nervous System Support

These herbs support the nervous system and dampen the effects of stress on the mood. Vitex supports low moods that are hormonal in origin.

- ½ ounce ashwagandha tincture

- ½ ounce vitex tincture

- ¼ ounce motherwort tincture

- ¼ ounce lemon balm tincture

- ¼ ounce skullcap tincture

- ¼ ounce passion flower tincture

Combine the above tinctures and store in an amber bottle. Take 2 ½ droppers or 1 teaspoon as needed, up to four times daily for 2 weeks. If symptoms persist or increase, please seek medical attention.

Gentle Night Tincture

A perfect "night cap" for those nights when your thoughts or worries keep you awake, rather than baby. I find this tincture is helpful when mothers find themselves having difficulty sleeping once baby has established a routine of nightly sleep.

- ¾ ounce passion flower tincture

- ½ ounce chamomile tincture

- ½ ounce skullcap tincture

- ¼ ounce lavender tincture

Combine the above tinctures and store in an amber bottle. Take 2 ½ droppers or 1 teaspoon as needed before bed or when you experience difficulty falling asleep with night wakings. If symptoms persist or increase, please seek medical attention.

Mother's Mood Lifter

One mother in my practice described this tincture as "a ray of sunshine breaking through the clouds."

- ½ ounce eleuthero tincture
- ½ ounce St John's wort tincture
- ¼ ounce licorice tincture
- ¼ ounce motherwort tincture
- ¼ ounce milky oats tincture
- ¼ ounce ginseng tincture

Combine the above tinctures and store in an amber bottle. Take 2 ½ droppers or 1 teaspoon twice daily for 3-4 weeks. Avoid taking in the late afternoon. If symptoms persist or increase, please seek medical attention. St John's wort is contraindicated if you are taking certain medications and can interfere with oral contraceptives. Licorice is contraindicated if you have high blood pressure.

Baby Blues Spray

Need to lift the mood quick? Spray this delightful concoction and make an instant shift in mood.

- 10 drops vanilla essential oil

- 10 drops tangerine essential oil

- 10 drops grapefruit essential oil

- 10 drops orange peel essential oil

Add drops to a spray bottle filled with filtered water. Shake and spray in your house whenever you need a boost.

These recommendations are not a substitute for meeting with a trained medical professional. If you are experiencing anxiety and/or depression, please seek help from a medical professional.

If you feel you're experiencing severe depression or if you have thoughts of hurting yourself or your baby, please see a medical professional immediately.

Getting help early can help you restore your mood and feel better sooner.

Placenta Encapsulation

Early in my pregnancy I remember attending a party where the subject of placenta encapsulation came up. Being the only pregnant women in the room, a woman I'd never met turned to me, with a disgusted look on her face and said, "I bet this conversation is totally grossing you out. You'd probably never want to eat your placenta." I laughed. "Of course I am going to eat my placenta!" I could tell by her face that she was shocked. "But there's no research to prove that it actually works," she said.

It's true that we have limited recent research on the subject of Placentophagia and most of what is reported is anecdotal. However, preparing and feeding the placenta to new mothers has been part of Chinese culture longer than modern medicine has existed.

" I decided to encapsulate my placenta with my second pregnancy. I had struggled with my mood and had such a hard time with my first child that I decided to try it. I am so happy I did. My mood was much more even, although I did cry often the first couple of weeks. I also felt like I had better energy and was able to keep up with my toddler and care for my baby. I wish I had done this with my first pregnancy. **~Anna, mother of two**

I believe there is a lot of wisdom found in the way cultures have traditionally cared for their mothers that science has yet to reveal, but are embraced and welcomed by mothers because they have witnessed the power in those traditions. Could it be placebo? Of course, placentophagia could be placebo, but I think there has been some evidence that has demonstrated the placenta does have medicinal value.

For example, in one study of 50 placentas, the average iron content of a placenta was found to be 75.5 mg, but some were as high as 170 mg.[1] When we birth, we lose blood and with it, we lose iron. Iron deficiency anemia can lead to fatigue and depression in new moms. Your placenta can be an excellent means to boost your mineral levels.

There is evidence in animal studies that the placenta contains Placental Opioid Enhancing Factor (POEF), which may reduce pain.[2,3]

In a 2013 study that surveyed 189 women, it was found that 95% of women who had consumed their placenta during their postpartum period reported a positive or very positive experience.[4]

* See Page 218 for Citations

Placenta consumption is believed to:

- Replenish iron stores

- Increase breast milk

- Reduce post-natal bleeding

- Balance your hormones

- Assist the uterus in returning to its pre-pregnancy state

- Increase energy

- Improve mood

What you should know about placenta encapsulation

Find someone who is experienced in placenta encapsulation. Some doulas and midwives perform this service.

The placenta should be refrigerated after it is birthed. It is important that you arrange how your placenta will be delivered to the person performing the encapsulation services so that your placenta does not go to waste.

The placenta will be prepared for encapsulation and may be steamed with traditional Chinese herbs or preped alone. Once dehydrated, it will be ground into a powder and placed in capsules. Placentas on average yield about 100-200 capsules.

Dosage varies widely with some experts recommending that you begin taking the capsules immediately and others advising that you wait until your milk comes in. Discuss dosage and timing with your midwife, OB or doula to ensure you are getting an individualized recommendation.

The capsules should be stored in a cool, dark place. Some women prefer to refrigerate them, which is preferable if you are in a warm climate.

Although most women report no taste at all, if you are concerned about taste then I would recommend storing in the refrigerator.

Currently, there is research being conducted and the first double-blind, controlled study may be published as early as 2016.

" My milk supply was low the first week and a half. The pediatrician was recommending formula, which I didn't want to do. My midwife suggested I stop my placenta pills and 2 days later my milk supply came in. She told me to start the placenta pills again and WOW, I was a walking milk machine after that. I think it was better for my body to start the placenta pills after my milk was in.

~Joyce, mother of two

HEALING YOUR THYROID & ADRENALS NATURALLY

Brief moments of panic flooded my mind and temporarily replaced the joy, peace, and contentment you embrace as a mother. Subtle enough to be attributed to the shift in hormones and lack of sleep every mom comes to know in those early months, I dismissed them.

Slowly, the dark mood crept in and the fatigue began to take hold of my life. I remember the days where it felt like I was fully submerged, trying to move, but the weight of each day would slow all progress.

I talked to doctors, not a doctor, but multiple doctors. The answer was the same—"Of course you're tired, you're a mom."

But as the days passed, my weight gain continued,

hair loss was now apparent, and my skin was beginning to resemble the scales of a reptile. My body hurt everywhere, all the time. And it progressively got worse. In the morning, I would cringe in anticipation of the searing pain of simply touching my foot to the ground.

Meanwhile, my doctor continued to say my labs looked fine and that I should reduce my stress.

But my labs didn't look fine and there were important markers I had requested that weren't ordered. My inflammation markers were elevated and for the first time in my life, I had elevated cholesterol levels.

I was doing everything right, wasn't I? I continued my prenatals, supported my adrenals, tried to exercise, slept well and ate an incredibly clean diet. I had tried elimination diets and optimized my gut for digestion but despite my efforts, nothing really budged.

One morning, after 15 hours of sleep, I fell asleep in front of my infant son at the breakfast table. My husband rushed to the kitchen in response to the baby's frantic screams. He shook me awake, insisting that my symptoms were definitely not normal. Like clues to an increasingly worrisome mystery, he began listing the manifestations of my postpartum ailment. In that moment I realized what was wrong—I was hypothyroid.

It had crept up so slowly and I shunned my inner voice so effectively in favor of following the "doctor's advice," I had missed the signs of hypothyroid altogether. Completely wrapped up in motherhood, work, and the crippling fatigue, I had neglected my own wisdom.

After ordering my own labs, it was evident I had developed postpartum thyroiditis and it had progressed into Hashimoto's thyroiditis. It was also evident that I was in need of thyroid medication.

Within a couple of months of taking the thyroid meds, I became pregnant, unexpectedly. Once again I found myself at the mercy of a doctor unwilling to order labs or treat my thyroid. Pregnancy is an interesting place to find yourself in when you're hypothyroid—most doctors aren't comfortable managing your thyroid and most midwives or OBs won't take you as a patient until you're at least 10 weeks pregnant—leaving a large gap in your care right when your baby is the most vulnerable.

This time, I ordered my own labs right away. But in need of a prescription, I was at the mercy of my doctor. I was denied the medication and referred to a midwife who wouldn't see me for several weeks. At this point, I desperately sought a second opinion, one that would offer me a much needed increase in my thyroid medication dose, but it was too late.

At 11 weeks, we lost the baby. Two weeks later, my symptoms were back with a vengeance. My heart was weighed down with grief, a grief my body was just too tired to support.

I would later come to find out, hypothyroidism was only one piece of my puzzle. I was now presenting with antibodies to my adrenals, connective tissue, as well as phospholipid antibodies. It was a lot to take in, especially as I continued to work and take care of my young son.

I cried. A lot.

But I refused to be a disease, a diagnosis or anything less than the woman and mother I yearned to be.

Every mother deserves to thrive. Every mother deserves to be heard.

I am grateful every day for my journey, for my experience as a patient and my struggles as mother. Through it all, a better version of me came to be. The birth of my son signaled the death of who I was and the rebirth of the woman, mother, and doctor I am today.

I've successfully managed my autoimmunity and have empowered mothers to do the same.

Autoimmune thyroid disease is often a subtle

condition when it initially presents. In the coming chapter, we'll discuss the symptoms and mechanisms behind the condition and why new mothers are at risk for developing postpartum thyroiditis.

Autoimmune Thyroid (Postpartum Thyroiditis)

Postpartum thyroiditis is one of the most common autoimmune conditions to affect new mothers. During postpartum thyroiditis the immune system attacks the thyroid, causing tissue destruction. In most women, postpartum thyroiditis begins with hyperthyroid (too much thyroid) symptoms following by hypothyroid (too little thyroid) symptoms. However, some women experience hypothyroid symptoms alone.

Symptoms of Hyperthyroidism:

- Anxiety or nervousness
- Difficulty sleeping or insomnia
- Weight loss
- Racing heart
- Shaking hands
- Inability to concentrate
- Loose stools

Symptoms of Hypothyroidism:

- Fatigue
- Depression
- Dry skin
- Hair loss
- Weight gain or difficulty losing weight
- Cold intolerance
- Memory loss or brain fog
- Headache
- Constipation
- Muscle aches and joint pain
- Reduction in breast milk supply
- Infertility

Pregnancy is considered a state of heightened immune tolerance. It's a common belief that the immune system is actually shut down or suppressed during pregnancy; however, this is not the case. What actually takes place is a down regulation of the aspect of the immune system that would recognize and attack baby (Th1) and a shift towards the part of the immune system what will allow for baby to develop in utero (Th2 dominance).

During pregnancy, we see the autoimmune conditions that are Th1 dominant tend to decrease and symptoms are suppressed. Following birth, these autoimmune conditions can reappear or become triggered. For some women, like myself, birth triggers the development of a new autoimmune condition.

The switch from Th2 dominance to Th1 dominance that occurs in the postpartum period is thought to be a trigger for postpartum thyroiditis since these autoantibodies, specifically the TPO antibodies, are induced by a Th1 mechanism. While postpartum thyroiditis is commonly associated with Th1 dominance, it is important to note that there are specific cases in which Th2 dominance can exist.

You are at higher risk for developing autoimmune thyroid disease during your postpartum period if you have a history of Hashimoto's thyroiditis, have a history of postpartum thyroiditis or have ever tested positive for anti-thyroid peroxidase or anti-thyroglobulin antibodies.

For many women, postpartum thyroiditis resolves in the first year postpartum, however even after resolution the condition may return. In about 20% of women the condition will persist and they will be diagnosed with Hashimoto's thyroiditis, an autoimmune thyroid condition.

" My mom has hypothyroid disease and I later found out that she struggled with postpartum depression only after mine became so bad. My mom went with me to the doctor and insisted that he test my thyroid. I was hypothyroid too. I didn't realize it was genetic and can come on after you have a baby. My mom has helped me in so many ways and without her I don't know if I would have come out of my depression.

~Kylie, mother of two

Because women who have had postpartum thyroiditis are at a higher risk of developing autoimmune thyroid later in life or with subsequent pregnancies, I recommend working with an experienced health care practitioner to address your condition holistically.

I've helped many postpartum women find relief from fatigue and autoimmunity in my practice. By screening for thyroid, adrenal and other underlying conditions, we are able to treat the root cause and restore thyroid function, while also preventing thyroid tissue destruction.

I recommend a complete thyroid panel be ordered if you suspect postpartum thyroiditis. This includes a TSH, Total T4, Free T4, Total T3, Free T3, Reverse T3, Anti-thyroglobulin antibodies,

Anti-thyroid peroxidase antibody and possibly Anti-thyroid receptor antibody. All too often, doctors will only order TSH, which measures how your brain is talking to your thyroid. TSH is only one portion of the picture and does not provide enough information to accurately evaluate your thyroid.

As a mother who personally struggled with postpartum thyroiditis, I am very passionate about screening mothers and making sure they get appropriate treatment for their thyroid condition. The right interventions applied early can reduce symptoms, protect your thyroid gland and help you avoid developing additional autoimmune conditions.

" Before my energy tanked I can remember being anxious after I had my daughter and thinking that was just normal. Then the fatigue hit and I could barely make it past bedtime routine. After a while my joints were painful and I was sick all the time. When I finally got thyroid treatment my energy returned and I felt so much better. I had no idea having a baby could cause a thyroid problem. **~Becky, mother of one**

Natural Remedies to Support Your Thyroid Health

Vitamin D3: 6,000 IU daily may help prevent and reverse autoimmune thyroid, while also supplying baby with the amount of vitamin D they need. I recommend patients achieve blood levels 60-70 nM when supplementing with vitamin D.

Selenium: 200 mcg daily may reduce inflammation and anti-TPO antibodies.

Prenatal Vitamins: Continue your prenatal, which will provide you with iron, B vitamins and iodine, which are all necessary for thyroid health.

Omega-3: 2,000-4,000 mg daily. EPA, like that found in fish oil, is an anti inflammatory and can help your immune system rebalance.

Probiotics: 25-50 billion daily, rotate strains every 4-6 weeks. Probiotics help modulate your immune system. Since the majority of your immune system is found in your gut, it is important that you support your gut health. I recommend advanced gut testing for many of my postpartum thyroid patients.

Turmeric: 1,000 mg twice daily. Curcumin, the active constituent of turmeric, is a potent anti-inflammatory and has been used in some cultures to increase breastmilk production. Turmeric can also be made into a tea (see page 164).

Eliminate Gluten: Gliadin, the protein portion of gluten, has an amino acid sequence that closely resembles the thyroid gland. When your immune system reacts to gluten, inflammation increases and through a process known as molecular mimicry, your body mistakenly attacks your thyroid.

To read more about gluten & thyroid disease visit: http://drbrighten.com/quit-gluten-now

" I never felt right after my son was born. I didn't take the time to go to the doctor because nothing I was experiencing was extreme, plus all of my friends and family were telling me it was normal. Two years later, I had my first miscarriage. I had 3 miscarriages before I found Dr. Brighten. She listened to my whole story and ordered testing. She discovered I had Hashimoto's and a gut infection. After working with her I felt better than I ever had and for the first time I felt deeply connected to my son. I was scared to try to have another baby and wasn't sure that I would. I'll never forget the fear and joy I experienced when to my surprise, my pregnancy test came back positive. I called Dr. Brighten right away. She helped me put together and plan and she supported me through my entire pregnancy. She also helped me plan for my postpartum time and with her help I felt much better this time around. My husband and I never thought we would have another baby. I am so blessed to have found Dr. Brighten and so grateful for her compassion. **~Melanie, mother of two**

Consider Elimination Diet: Food sensitivities can contribute to and cause autoimmune symptoms to become worse. An elimination diet can help you identify foods that may be a trigger for you. I recommend breastfeeding moms work with an experienced practitioner who can help them identify problematic foods while also ensuring they are receiving all the nutrients they and their baby need.

Avoid Toxins: BPA, heavy metals, fluoride and other chemicals stress the body and negatively impact thyroid health. They can also lead to leaky gut, which can make autoimmunity worse. Visit www.EWG.org to understand how you can avoid chemicals in your environment.

Support Your Adrenals: Your adrenal glands help control the inflammation in your body and assist proper thyroid function. (See page 122)

In my online program, *The Seed & The Soil: Hashimoto's Guide to Fertility*, we take women through a thorough elimination diet and help them heal themselves from autoimmune thyroid disease. During this program, I share the therapies I've used with hundreds of women to help them put their autoimmunity into remission and enhance their fertility. If you are interested in learning more please visit: **http://drbrighten.com/seedandsoil**

Thyroid Medication

Some women require thyroid medication based on their symptoms and lab results. If your thyroid symptoms persist longer than a year, it is possible you will require lifelong thyroid medication. By working to put your autoimmunity into remission, you can prevent further thyroid destruction and may be able to eliminate or reduce your medication dosage.

The most common synthetic thyroid medication includes Synthroid (Levothyroxine) and is what most conventional doctors will prescribe for hypothyroidism. Synthroid is a synthetic T4 that relies on the body for conversion to T3, the active hormone. However, if you are having issues converting T4 to T3, perhaps due to nutritional deficiencies or chronic stress, you are unlikely to benefit from this medication. Cytomel (Liothyronine) is a synthetic T3 and may be given in addition to Synthroid or alone.

Some individuals may not tolerate synthetic thyroid, which may be due to their body reacting to the binders and fillers in the medications. In these cases, having a compounded thyroid medication may be a better option.

Iodine & Postpartum Thyroiditis

Iodine is generally not recommended in autoimmune thyroid conditions because it may cause an increase in symptoms, especially when a woman is low in selenium. It is important to work with an experienced health care practitioner who can help you understand if iodine supplementation is right for you. All pregnant women should receive iodine as it is necessary for baby's development.

Compounded formulas of T4 and T3, made from scratch at a special compounding pharmacy are often best for patients who react poorly to both synthetically and naturally derived thyroid because the ratios of T4 and T3 can be adjusted to fit your body and can also be made without superfluous fillers that may trigger autoimmunity. Using this option, you can also have sustained-release compounded medication, to allow for a slower absorption.

It is important to find a high quality compounding pharmacy to ensure that every dose of medication contains the same amount of T4 and T3 every time. Your doctor should be able to recommend a pharmacy that uses high quality materials and avoids the use of potentially allergenic fillers.

Naturally derived thyroid is a combination of both T4 and T3. Most people have heard of Armour Thyroid, but other common brands are Nature-Thyroid and West Thyroid Pure. Many patients report doing better on these because they offer a combination of hormones, which means you are relying less on the body's ability to convert T4 to T3.

It is important to note that, while it is rare, some patients have antibodies to not only their thyroid, but to the hormones themselves. In these situations you may find that naturally-derived thyroid hormone makes you feel much worse than when taking a synthetic hormone or even no hormone at all. That doesn't mean there's anything wrong with you and there is no *right or wrong* as far as medications goes. Instead, we just need to figure out what works for you, which medication makes you feel your best, and what is really helping control (not just cover up) your condition.

              I felt like I was in slow motion all the time. My brain was slow, my body was slow and no matter how much I slept I was just so tired. My doctor kept telling me to get more help at home. When I finally got him to order a thyroid test he said my TSH was the highest he'd ever seen! **~Tamara, mother of two**

Follow-up Testing

Once you've began thyroid medication, it's important to follow up with a blood test approximately four to six weeks after you are on a consistent dose A "consistent dose" means that your doctor hasn't changed your prescription at all during that time. Your test results should be evaluated in conjunction with your symptoms to determine if the dose is appropriate. Just because your thyroid labs look normal doesn't mean you'll be symptom-free. If you are experiencing symptoms or if you feel worse when you began a medication, it's very important to contact your prescribing physician.

It's important to become educated about the different thyroid medications available to you, but taking thyroid medication unsupervised can yield negative consequences. I never recommend beginning a medication without your doctor's direct supervision.

Postpartum Depression and Thyroid

If your doctor has diagnosed you with postpartum depression, I highly recommend having your thyroid tested. Hypothyroidism may be the root cause of your depression.

Adrenal Dysfunction

You've probably heard the term "adrenal fatigue." It is a term used to describe a collection of symptoms that arise from disruption in adrenal function, which may be due to issues with the hypothalamus, pituitary, or adrenal glands and how they communicate.

But the term adrenal fatigue can be a bit misleading because in most cases your adrenals glands aren't actually fatigued or tired. Instead, there is a disruption of the Hypothalamic-Adrenal-Pituitary axis (HPA), essentially the way in which your brain and adrenals are communicating.

To give a brief overview, when we experience stress (baby crying, skipping a meal, work deadlines, etc.), the hypothalamus in our brain releases corticotropin releasing factor (CRF), which signals the pituitary to release adrenocorticotropic hormone (ACTH). ACTH's job is to signal the adrenal glands to secrete cortisol, epinephrine, and norepinephrine.

The disruption in the HPA axis can occur under times of prolonged stress, but can also be a result of going through childbirth.

For new mothers, adrenal fatigue symptoms can come on more suddenly due to the huge amount of stress from birth and bringing a new infant home. In mothers, adrenal fatigue often presents itself as increased sensitivity to stress or difficulty coping with stress. Feeling overwhelmed by day-to-day life, exhausted, agitated, or anxious about the slightest events may be a clue that your adrenals are struggling.

What does adrenal dysfunction look like?

- Difficulty waking in the morning

- Afternoon fatigue

- Craving sugar, salt, or fat

- Increased illness due to immune system depression

- Hormone imbalance

- Acne and other skin problems

- Depression

- Low libido

- Poor memory

- Increased PMS and menopausal symptoms

- Dizziness, feeling light headed or "head rush" when rising from lying or seated

- Irritability

- Inability to cope with stress

How are the adrenals tested?

Most doctors will only test a morning cortisol and maybe ACTH, which signals the release of cortisol. I recommend that you have at least a four-point salivary cortisol collection to determine your daily output. A 21-hydroxylase antibody testing should be considered if you have a family history of autoimmunity or have abnormal cortisol findings as this may be a sign of Addison's disease.

A common test used in Functional and Naturopathic Medicine to assess adrenal health is the Adrenal Stress Index (ASI) test. An ASI looks at six parameters in evaluating your adrenal health.

1. Four Cortisol Measurements: Helps evaluate your stress response and your rhythm of cortisol release during the day.

2. Insulin: Evaluates blood sugar regulation.

3. DHEA: Helps determine how you've adapted to stress.

4. Secretory IgA: Evaluates impact on the immune system and gut permeability.

5. 17-OH Progesterone: Helps determine adrenal reserve.

6. Gluten antibodies: Helps determine intolerance to gluten.

Natural Remedies to Support Your Adrenal Health

Breastfeed & Cuddle Your Baby. Oxytocin, the hormone that is released when you breastfeed and cuddle your little one protects your body from the negative effects of stress.

Be Gentle with Yourself. You are one wonderful woman and you are doing an amazing job. Please, remember this as often as possible. Being a mom is hard and being gentle with yourself is important.

Eat Regularly. Consume regular meals, not allowing yourself to go long periods without eating. Low blood sugar is hard on the adrenals.

Eat Protein with Every Meal. This will support healthy blood sugar levels and allow your body to relax, knowing that it has plenty of fuel.

Include Carbohydrates. Limiting carbohydrates to less than 20% of your caloric intake can be metabolically stressful for your body, especially when you're breastfeeding.

Probiotics. Take a 25 billion CFU multistrain probiotic daily or consume fermented foods such as sauerkraut, homemade yogurt, kombucha, or kefir. Healthy gut bacteria promote adrenal health. When underlying gut infections are present, the adrenal glands can become overworked. Work with an experienced practitioner to investigate if your gut health is contributing to adrenal fatigue.

Lower Stress. Breathe deeply and often, meditate, practice mindfulness in the moments you can, and please honor your strength. Take note of what you have to be grateful for.

Sleep. Ask your partner to take the children on the weekend so you can sleep in or take a nap. Go to bed by 10 p.m. most nights and sleep in a completely dark room.

Exercise. Strength training, gentle cardio, and stretching are best for adrenal health. Long cardio routines and strenuous exercise can often make adrenal conditions worse. Meet with a health care provider to determine the right type of exercise for your health needs. Often, daily exercise that is at your level will help improve your energy and mood.

Rhodiola rosea. 30-60 drops of tincture 2-3 times daily. I call this the endurance herb because it supports both mental and physical stamina. Rhodiola improves energy, lowers anxiety, reduces inflammation and supports your immune system. It should not be taken if you have a history of bipolar depression.

Ashwagandha. 30 drops of tincture 3 times daily. Ashwagandha improve energy and memory while also reducing anxiety. It improves immune system function and lowers inflammation. Ashwagandha also supports thyroid health. If you have a sensitivity to nightshades, you may not tolerate Ashwagandha as it is in the same family.

Tulsi or Holy Basil. 30-60 drops of tincture 2-3 times daily. This herb reduces fatigue and can help elevate mood in cases of mild depression.

Eleutherococcus or Siberian ginseng. Start with 20 drops of tincture twice daily before 12 pm. Eleuthero increases energy, your ability to concentrate and mental alertness. It can be overstimulating for some people which is why I recommend starting with 20 drops of tincture to see how you feel first. This herb should be avoided if you have high blood pressure.

Magnesium Glycinate. 150-300 mg nightly. Magnesium supports adrenal gland function.

B-Complex. Specifically, pantothenic acid (B5) and pyridoxine (B6) are necessary for proper adrenal function. Pantothenic acid is necessary for adrenal structural integrity, while pyridoxine is important for cortisol production. I recommend supplementing with a B complex rather than specific B vitamins to avoid creating B vitamin depletion.

Vitamin C. 2,000-4,000 mg daily. Your adrenal glands require vitamin C to synthesize hormones. It is better to have vitamin C in whole foods than ascorbic acid.

Power Pose. Stand with your hands on your hips and feet in a wide stance. Feel your feet firmly planted in the ground and take five long breaths. Spending 2-3 minutes in this pose can help lower your stress response. As mothers, we are often in positions that cause our body to be closed in (shoulders rounded in, arms cross body as you hold your infant). Making a conscious effort to open up and expand into your space can help lower your body's perception of stress.

If you suspect you have adrenal fatigue, please consult with an experienced health care practitioner to ensure you receive proper testing and treatment.

" Every little thing and I mean, every little thing would make me want to blow up. I was either yelling or crying. Once I started herbs and vitamins for my adrenals my mood improved, but it wasn't until I began meditating that I finally felt like myself again. I think it's funny I didn't see that the answer to my chaos was to sit quietly. **~Sara, mother of three**

MAMA SELF CARE

"A woman's creative essence provides her with infinite resources."

—Tami Lynn Kent

When you have a baby, it is the end of the person you once knew and the beginning of you as a mother. In a way, the birth of your child also signals the birth of you as mother. And in these following months you can choose how to define yourself and reinvent that as many times as you'd like.

The unfortunate reality is, as you enter into motherhood, our society asks that you relinquish any idea of autonomy—any idea of being anything more than a mother. However, it's important that you continue to seek out the things that bring joy to your life and that you set time aside to really focus on how you want to define yourself. Yes, you're a mother, but that isn't where the definition of you as a whole person ends.

You must tend to yourself. Your child demands that you are present, which makes the temptation to disconnect from yourself at the end of a long day much more tempting.

When I was in the thick of it in the early weeks postpartum, I'd roll out my yoga mat and take a savasana (corpse pose). As I lay there I would envision the earth coming up to meet me. Letting my weight sink in, I visualized the great Mother Earth's energy holding me up. In that moment I was grounded and I felt supported. I recommend this to women in my practice and would encourage you to try sinking into Mother Earth's supportive energy, especially when you feel tempted to disconnect.

Engaging Your Creative Center

Your pelvis is the home of your sacral chakra and your creative energy. When you are tapped into this space you have the ability to be more creative with problem solving the challenges that arise.

Sacral Chakra Meditation:

1. Coming into a comfortable seated position, feel the weight of your sit bones on the earth. Visualizing the tailbone as a root, let it drop down and connect into the earth.

2. Placing your hands over your womb space, close your eyes and begin to send your breath into your pelvis. At first, observe without judgment of what comes up as you begin to explore this space.

3. As you breathe, visualize that earth energy drawing up into the pelvis. Let it swirl and fill your space.

4. Placing an imaginary filter above your head, draw in a beautiful golden light and let it meet that earth energy in your pelvis. Allow them to swirl, connect, and integrate.

5. Imagine this energy washing through the pelvis, allowing anything that is not

serving you to drop down that root and surrender it to the earth.

6. This is your space, fill it with what you desire in your life and release anything that you no longer wish to keep.

To close, visualize closing off the light energy and releasing all to the highest good. Take a final deep breath and as you exhale, bow forward. Inhale and on the exhale return to seated.

Feel like you have no time for this?

At any time you can simply place a hand on the front of your pelvis and another on your back, just over the sacrum. Send your awareness into this space, even if just briefly. By building this connection you strengthen your ability to drop into a grounded space when life becomes hectic or stressful.

As women, we can store a lot of past grief or traumas that can be released or ignited with birth. Meeting with a pelvic floor therapist or intuitive counselor can help you transition and process the shifts that have evolved after childbirth.

If you are interested in exploring more of the energetics of mothering, I highly recommend the book, *Mothering from Your Center* by Tami Lynn Kent. She has been a mentor of mine and taught me the art and skill of Holistic Pelvic Care™.

Are you meeting your basic needs?

Give yourself one point for each of the following:

_____   I eat regular meals and avoid skipping meals and snacks.

_____   I take the time to chew my food well.

_____   I rest often, especially when I feel tired.

_____   I drink fluids throughout the day.

_____   I move my body regularly.

_____   I sleep in a dark room.

_____   I spend time in the sunshine at least 3 days per week.

_____   I cuddle, hug, or engage in physical touch daily.

_____   I am gentle, loving, and forgiving with myself.

_____   I make time for a shower or bath most days of the week.

_____   : Total

If you find yourself with a score of 7 or less, it is time to recruit some help and make a strategy to meet these needs. You are an important an integral part of your family and friends' lives. You must take care of your own health if you are going to be 100% present for those who you care for.

Beyond the basics, you deserve to thrive.

It is not indulgent to care for yourself. Repeat. It is not indulgent to care for yourself, to spend time doing the things you enjoy or to take a break to fill your heart with joy.

Life is more than feedings, naps, burping, diaper changes...you get the idea. It is easy to slip into the role of mom and forget that you are a woman with needs. You will be so much happier if you focus on staying connected with those things that bring you joy. And you'll be a better mom too!

As a working mom, I know all to well how difficult it can be to make time for yourself. I want to share with you a few of my favorite "mini-spa" rituals that I use when I need a little pampering, but am short on time.

" Why do moms feel so guilty about taking 'me time?' I didn't think I deserved or could afford to take time for myself. It took my third child for me to realize that there was no way I would make it through my days anymore unless I started to make more time for what I loved. It wasn't easy, but it was necessary. **~Jacklyn, mother of three**

What about going back to work?

Studies have shown that if mother goes to work and that's what makes her happy, baby is happier and better adjusted. If mom stays home and that makes her happy, then baby is happy and better adjusted as well. All of this is to say, you need to make this decision for yourself.

It is important for you to listen to what's right for you and to know that you can change your mind at any time. Just because you decided to go back to work doesn't mean you need to continue working (as long as finances aren't an issue). If that isn't working for your family, then I encourage you to look at alternatives. Maybe you go to part time, maybe you find a new job, maybe you quit working altogether.

If you decided you want to be a stay-at-home mom and that is a struggle for you, look at ways to work outside the home or even work within your home. Maybe you can pick up a hobby that would fill that need and that desire to work. Whatever it is, don't compare yourself to anyone else, to any other mother, and certainly not to your mother. You are your own individual, your own person, and it is for you to define how you will mother your child.

When Sleep Isn't Enough

You've probably heard it multiple times—"sleep when baby sleeps." This is great advice, but sometimes, sleeping when baby sleeps isn't enough.

Exhaustion, low mood, anxiety, joint pain, and cold hands and feet are likely signs of larger underlying issues. Hypothyroidism, adrenal fatigue, B12 deficiency anemia, iron deficiency anemia, and autoimmune disease may be contributing to your symptoms.

If you feel like your fatigue goes beyond what should be expected in motherhood you should speak with your doctor to have a thorough workup. With an exam, complete history and proper laboratory work, your doctor should be able to identify the cause of your exhaustion.

Autoimmunity, a condition in which your immune system mistakenly attacks your own body tissue, can be triggered by childbirth. The symptoms are often difficult to differentiate and may wax and wane for many months and sometimes years. It is important that you seek help from a qualified medical professional who is willing to listen to your story and partner with you to understand what is the cause of your symptoms.

If you suspect something is wrong, don't delay care. Trust your instincts. Addressing autoimmunity early can help you prevent the development of more serious conditions.

Natural Remedies to Increase Energy

Nutritional Supplementation. If you are found to be low in iron, vitamin B12, or other nutrients your fatigue will be amplified. Continuing your prenatal vitamins can help guard against deficiencies, but blood work may be necessary to determine if you have a deficiency or anemia.

Legs Up the Wall (Viparita Karani). This simple yoga pose can be incredibly rejuvenating. Sit close to a wall with the right side of your body touching. As you begin to lay down, allow your legs to move up the wall until they are resting comfortably against it. You can also place a pillow or bolster under your hips to add support.

Rest Often. More than just sleep, whenever possible put your feet up and relax.

Eat Well, Eat Often. Skipping meals or eating processed foods and added, processed sugar will cause your energy to crash and trigger hormone imbalance.

Nurse with Baby Near. Co-sleeping or having a bassinet near your bed can make night feedings less disruptive to your sleep.

Accept Help. Having a baby is a lot of work. If someone offers help, please accept it. There is no shame in not being able to do it all. No one should have to do it all.

Ask for Help. If you need help, you need help. The only way your loved ones will know how to best help you is for you to let them know what you need.

Be Gentle with Yourself. Negative thoughts about your abilities or your life are draining. You're doing an awesome job and even when it doesn't feel that way, please be gentle with yourself.

Be a Team. You and your partner need to communicate and work together. If you don't have someone you are partnering with, I urge you consider hiring a postpartum doula or connecting with someone else in your life that can help you.

Avoid Dehydration. Staying hydrated has numerous benefits, including sustained energy.

Choose Healthy Snacks. When you are feeling low, chocolate, potato chips, and easy energy dense foods sound pretty appealing. However, any boost in energy they provide is temporary and you will crash.

Go For a Walk. Yes, I know this seems like a strange recommendation, but even a short gentle walk can help raise your energy and mood.

Fix Nutrient Deficiencies. Vitamin B12, iron, vitamin D, and other nutrients can be tested for and supplemented if necessary.

Ashwagandha Tincture. 2 droppers full twice daily as needed for a pick me up.

I cannot express enough how important it is to address the root cause of your fatigue. If your fatigue is due to a deeper issue, these practices will be helpful, but will not be enough to properly restore your energy and vitality.

Gentle Energy Lifting Tea

Gotu kola and licorice support healthy energy, while the other supporting herbs in this tea feed and nourish your tissues, especially the adrenals.

Ingredients

- ½ ounce gotu kola leaf
- ½ ounce nettle leaf
- ½ ounce red raspberry leaf
- ¼ ounce licorice root
- ¼ ounce yellow dock

Directions

Place all ingredients in a bowl and mix. Store in a mason jar.

To brew a cup of tea: Steep 1 tablespoon of herbs in 1 cup of hot water for 10 minutes, covered.

To brew a large batch: Steep 4 tablespoons of herbs per quart of boiling water for 30 minutes.

Drink 1-4 cups daily.

Homemade Self Care Recipes

Lavender Body Scrub

This is one of my favorite scrubs to use at the end of a long day. I often use it as a facial exfoliator before bed.

Ingredients

- 1 cup sea salt
- ½ cup olive oil
- 10-15 drops lavender essential oil

Directions

Combine ingredients and store in a clean container.

To Use

Massage into skin using a gentle, circular motion during a shower or onto face before bed. Rinse well and pat dry.

Invigorating Salt Scrub

Grapefruit scent is an instant mood and energy pick me up. I especially love using this scrub on my hands during the winter months when they are dry and I could use a little perk.

Ingredients

- 1 cup sea salt
- ½ cup coconut oil
- 5 drops grapefruit essential oil

Directions

Combine ingredients and store in a clean container.

To Use

Massage into skin using a gentle, circular motion during a shower or onto face before bed. Rinse well and pat dry.

Vanilla Sugar Scrub

This is like a warm cookie for your skin. No seriously! Every time I use this I have that same warm feeling inside that I get when I smell fresh baked cookies. It's comforting.

Ingredients

- 2 cups brown sugar
- 1 cup coconut oil
- 1 teaspoon vanilla extract

Directions

Place all the ingredients into a food processor and whip until it is smooth and similar to cookie dough consistency.

Store in a cool location to keep oil from separating. If oil separates, stir with a spoon or even your finger.

To Use

Massage into skin using a gentle, circular motion during a shower or onto face before bed. Rinse well and pat dry.

Coffee Scrub

I pretty much love coffee everything! Something about that smell just gets me. In my early months I didn't drink coffee, but would enjoy this scrub. The coffee and oils are rejuvenating for the skin.

Ingredients

- ¼ cup coconut oil
- ⅓ cup coconut sugar
- 3 tablespoons fresh ground coffee (no imitation coffee)
- ¼ teaspoon cinnamon

Directions

Mix all ingredients well until a smooth mixture forms.

To Use

Massage into skin using a gentle, circular motion during a shower or onto face before bed. Rinse well and pat dry.

Baby Body Butter

The oils and butters in this cream deeply moisturize and repairs skin. You skin will be soft, plump and well hydrated when using this cream. I used this throughout my pregnancy to prevent stretch marks and after to help them heal.

Ingredients

- 2 ounces raw shea butter
- 2 ounces Nourishing Calendula Salve (see page 12)
- 1 tablespoon almond oil
- 1 teaspoon vitamin E oil
- 5 drops lavender or other oil (optional)

Directions

Place all the ingredients in a bowl. Using a mixer whip using until it is a smooth consistency.

To Use

Apply liberally

Refreshing Minty Lime Foot Bath

This is a wonderful little pick me up.

Ingredients

- 1 cup Epsom salt
- ¼ cup baking soda
- 3-4 drops lime essential oil (if making for an immediate soak, use juice from ½ lime)
- 5 drops peppermint essential oil

Directions

Mix ingredients thoroughly

To Use

Add ½ cup to a basin of warm water. Stir to dissolve. Soak feet when it has reached the ideal temperature.

Quick Eye Soothing Remedy

When I've had one of those inevitable sleepless nights, this is a quick trick I use to soothe my tired eyes.

Directions

Take two chamomile tea bags and steep in hot water for about 5 minutes. Take the bags out and place on a plate. Allow them to cool just enough to be tolerated over the eyes (drink the tea while you wait). Place the one tea bag over each eye and relax for the next 5 minutes.

NOURISHING YOUR BODY: NUTRITION FOR NEW MOMS

Your nutrition is just as important after birth as it was during pregnancy. It may be tempting to jump into a diet as soon as possible with the hopes of losing weight and regaining your pre-baby body. However, I strongly urge you to focus less on weight loss and more on rebuilding your nutrient stores and supplying the most nutrient-dense breast milk to your baby.

I know it's hard to have the extra weight your body gained during pregnancy without the adorable baby bump on the front to go with it. But that weight actually serves a purpose—it protects you and serves as an energy storehouse for you and baby.

So while there's nothing wrong with wanting to regain your pre-baby body, we're going to focus instead on optimizing every cell in your body.

Breastfeeding your infant places higher caloric energy and nutrient demands on your body. Your body is providing fuel to a quickly growing human. Your baby is growing faster and is moving more than they were in the womb, which means they need more nutrition from you. The recommended intake for micronutrients is based on what is excreted through your breast milk, although your needs may be higher if you have an underlying condition or are healing from a very traumatic birth.

What if I'm Not Breastfeeding?

There are a number of reasons why a woman may not breastfeed. If you are not breastfeeding, you still require a diet of high-quality foods to help you body heal and to prevent issues from arising.

On a separate, but related note, your relationship with breastfeeding is between you and your baby. Sure, we all know that breast milk is best, but it doesn't always work out for every mom. Be gentle with yourself.

The estimated additional caloric needs for a breastfeeding woman are about 500 to 700 more calories per day. Focus on eating highly nutrient-dense foods and less on counting calories. If you are severely restricting calories in an effort to lose weight you will not only compromise your milk supply, but also create stress on your body, which can result in hormonal imbalances and an inability to lose weight. For daily nutrient requirements for lactation vs. pregnancy, see the Appendix B (see page 205).

Nutrition Necessities for Healthy Mom and Baby

- Eat when you're hungry.

- Choose nutrient-dense foods; avoid "junk" or processed foods. When in doubt, avoid food in packaging.

- Eat protein and fat with every meal.

- Don't skip meals.

- Carry snacks with you.

- Ask a friend to make a meal delivery registry for you.

- Aim for 6-10 servings of vegetables daily.

Hydration

For most postpartum women, drinking at least 80 ounces of water a day is necessary to ensure they are staying adequately hydrated. One of the obvious reasons to stay hydrated is to support breast milk production. Dehydration can create a drop in milk supply, which is both frustrating and emotionally draining.

The Problem with Dehydration

Dehydration causes a hormone called *arginine vasopressin* (AVP) to be released, which in turn constricts blood vessels and causes water retention. AVP also signals cortisol release from the adrenals. Over time, the adrenal glands can become fatigued and other hormones will become disrupted, such as thyroid and progesterone.

Dehydration can also cause a decline in brain function, headaches, put you at risk for urinary tract infections, and cause hormonal disruption, so make sure that you're getting plenty of water.

Drinking all of that water may sound a little daunting to you. Eating soups, homemade popsicles or "spa water" infused with fruits or vegetables can provide you with additional fluids.

The Secret Mama's Super Food

Offal is one of the best kept secrets for helping a new mother heal. What is offal? Offal is the term used to describe organ meats. Now before you make up your mind, hear me out.

Organ meats have been consumed by many cultures for thousands of years. These same cultures recognize how incredibly nutrient-dense organ meats are and have served them to women after childbirth to help them heal for generations.

Feeling Squeamish About Liver? Try This Trick!

Cut raw liver into pieces small enough to swallow. Place the pieces in a freezer bag and place flat in the freezer. Be sure not to overcrowd the bad so that the pieces are easy to separate later. After 2-3 weeks in the freezer, swallow 2-3 liver pieces daily for the first 6 weeks postpartum.

Be sure to freeze for at least 2 weeks to kill any harmful organisms that may be present.

❝ I thought Dr. Brighten was crazy when she told me to eat liver. I didn't think there was anyway I'd be able to do it or that it was going to help my anemia after everything I had tried. A few months in and I not only felt better, but actually enjoyed the taste.

~Susan, mother of one

Eating organ meats provides the body with the necessary nutrients to repair damaged tissue, support the immune system, and provide essential nutrients to baby, such as vitamin A. If you're not ready to try organ meat, consuming bone broth or gelatin provides many nutrients and is much more versatile.

❝ I tell all my friends about bone broth. I stocked my freezer with it before I had my daughter and drank at least ½ cup a day for the first 2 months after she was born. My body healed really well and I felt strong. I know the bone broth helped.

~Tanya, mother of two

Noble Nutrients in Organ Meats

Organ Meat	Notable Nutrients
Liver	High source active vitamin A. Iron, copper, potassium, vitamin B12, magnesium, phosphorous, manganese, folate, choline
Heart	CoQ10, zinc, B vitamins, selenium, and iron.
Bone Broth	Glycine, glutamine, arginine, calcium, magnesium, potassium, phosphorus
Gelatin/ Collagen	An array of amino acids that help to rebuild and reinforce connective tissues and promote healing.

Nutrition to Help You Heal

Leafy Green Vegetables

Leafy greens are an excellent source of fiber, which will help keep your bowels regular, facilitate the removal of waste from your body and supports healthy hormones. They also provide an array of nutrients, including antioxidants, calcium and folate. The vitamin C, vitamin A, beta carotene they contain supports tissue healing.

Eating 2-3 cups of leafy greens daily will not only provide your body with the nutrients it needs to heal, but will also enrich your breast milk and can increase your breast milk supply. Take note however, if you eat 3 or more cups you may find your breast milk has a green tint. This isn't a sign that anything is wrong with your breastmilk, but quite the opposite— it is a sign of nutrient dense milk.

Fermented Foods

Foods like kefir, kombucha, kvass, sauerkraut and homemade yogurt provide your gut with beneficial bacteria. These bacteria promote healthy digestion and immune function. Since approximately 70% or more of your immune system is found in your gut, optimizing your gut health is one of the best ways to ensure a strong immune system.

Your digestive tract is also responsible for absorbing nutrients and those healthy gut bugs even produce some of your nutrients. When your gut is functioning at its best it will also ensure the removal of metabolic waste and toxins from the system. There are a lot of reasons to care for your gut and eating fermented foods is an easy way to nourish the system.

Aim for 3 tablespoons of fermented vegetables, 3-4 ounces of fermented beverages or ½-1 cup of yogurt daily. If you do not tolerate dairy you can opt for water kefir, coconut kefir, or coconut yogurt.

Pastured Ghee or Butter

Not only do these provide you with the fat your body needs to fuel your brain and breast milk supply, but they are also rich in important nutrients to help your body heal. Vitamins A, D, E and K2 are necessary for healing your skin and in support bone re-mineralization. It is also a source of minerals that support thyroid and adrenal health, which include selenium, iodine, zinc and copper.

Omega-3 Fatty Acid

Your baby's brain is developing rapidly and the fat you eat impacts their cognitive development. It also impacts your brain. Your brain shrinks up to 8% in the third trimester and it doesn't recover until about 6 months postpartum. Wow, right?

DHA is an omega-3 that feeds the brain. EPA is another form of omega-3 that lowers inflammation and has positive effects on both the brain and body.

Aim for three servings of omega-3 rich foods per week. Animal sources are easier for the body to utilize, as we are inefficient at converting plant sources into active forms. I recommend sardines, salmon, mackerel, and anchovies as excellent sources of omega-3s.

Mercury contamination is an issue in larger fish. I recommend The Monterey Bay Aquarium's Seafood Watch website to determine which fish are the lowest in mercury. www.seafoodwatch.org

If you choose to supplement with DHA and EPA I recommend a quality fish oil. Purchase from a reputable company that uses Good Manufacturing Practices and third party testing.

There are vegetarian forms derived from algae, but you will need to take a lot more to get an adequate amount.

Vitamin D

Vitamin D is an important nutrient for everyone, but especially nursing moms. Vitamin D enables you to absorb calcium, improves immunity and protects against certain chronic diseases. Your baby depends on you for vitamin D.

The majority of vitamin D is synthesized in your skin as it is exposed to sunlight. Getting a daily dose of sunshine has many benefits, but depending on where you are in the world or if you have darker skin, you may not be able to synthesize all that your body requires. Before supplementing, have your levels tested to determine if you need a supplement and how much.

Iron

Continuing your prenatal and eating iron rich food should provide you with all the iron your body needs during the next 6 weeks. However, if you had very heavy bleeding or continue to bleed heavily please check in with your doctor to ensure you to do not become anemic. A simple blood test called a CBC can determine if you are anemic and an iron panel can help you assess your current stores.

Anemia can affect your mood, energy, and overall health.

" After the birth of my son I was completely exhausted. People tell you you'll be tired, but you really have no idea until you literally stop sleeping. But in my case, I was so exhausted that walking up a flight of stairs caused complete exhaustion and left me out of breath. I just thought I was out of shape. When I went to my doctor for annual check up they told me I had iron deficiency anemia. I had stopped taking my prenatal a few months after my son was born. I started an iron supplement and within a few months my energy was back. ~**Julia, mother of one**

AFTERWARD

Being a mother is one of the most amazing and challenging experiences you will have in this life. Everyday you will learn more about who you are and what you are capable of. And you will find that you are capable of quite a bit.

As mothers, we find ourselves trying to do it all. I'm guilty of this and am always striving to find my balance in life. I remind myself, "It's a dance." But even in the midst of that dance it is easy to lose track of who is leading or what the next move may be.

When you inevitably find yourself fumbling, try to find your inner stillness and return to that which brings you joy. It is so easy to get caught up in all there is to do as a mother and to care for a family that you may very well find that this new life has left no space for your needs and desires.

Take care not to lose yourself in this journey. The happiest and most fulfilled of mothers are neither perfect nor have they relinquished their identity and appetite for a joy filled life. Your ability to mother depends on your ability to meet your needs and care for yourself.

Please be kind and gentle. This journey is filled with light, but the terrain varies wildly.

Take a deep breath—you've got this.

APPENDIX A: RECIPES

Turmeric Ginger Tea

Turmeric and ginger are wonderful herbs for decreasing inflammation, soothing your digestive tract and gently warming the body. Enjoy this tea any time of day!

Ingredients

- 1 teaspoon fresh grated ginger
- 1 teaspoon fresh grated turmeric
- 1-2 cups of water
- Raw honey to sweeten

Directions

Simmer herbs and water together for 10 minutes. Strain herbs and add honey to sweeten.

Nutritive Mother's Milk Tea

Rich with minerals and vitamin C, this tea provides nutrients that support a new mother's body and help to increase milk supply. The chamomile and fennel also relieve abdominal gas and bloating.

Ingredients

- 1 ounce blessed thistle leaves

- 1 ounce red raspberry leaves

- 1 ounce dried nettle leaves

- 1 ounce chamomile flowers

- 1 ounce dandelion leaf

- $\frac{1}{4}$ ounce fennel seeds

- $\frac{1}{2}$ ounce rose hips

Directions

Place all ingredients in a bowl and mix. Store in a mason jar.

To brew a cup of tea: Steep 1 tablespoon of herbs in 1 cup of hot water for 10 minutes, covered.

To brew a large batch: Steep 4 tablespoons of herbs per quart of boiling water for 30 minutes.

Drink 1-4 cups daily.

You can enjoy with a small amount honey too!

Calming Mother's Milk Tea

I find this tea to be really lovely before a nap or at bedtime to help relax the mind and body. The combination of catnip, chamomile, lemon balm and lavender calm the nerves and offer a sweet little cup of bliss.

Ingredients

- 1 ounce blessed thistle leaves

- 1 ounce fenugreek

- 1 ounce red raspberry leaves

- 1 ounce catnip

- 1 ounce chamomile flowers

- 1 ounce lemon balm

- ⅛ ounce lavender flowers

Directions

Place all ingredients in a bowl and mix. Store in a mason jar.

To brew a cup of tea: Steep 1 tablespoon of herbs in 1 cup of hot water for 10 minutes, covered.

To brew a large batch: Steep 4 tablespoons of herbs per quart of boiling water for 30 minutes.

Drink 1-4 cups daily.

If you want to enjoy a relaxing tea without boost breast milk, leave out the blessed thistle and fenugreek.

Fenugreek can be a little overpowering for some women to drink as a tea. You can always take fenugreek capsules instead if this is true for you.

Restorative Mother's Milk Tea

Licorice and ashwagandha help the body rebalance and support glands, such as the thyroid. Milky oats are considered a nervine, which is another way of saying it nourishes and calms the nervous system. The herbs in this tea blend support a healthy mood, energy, and stamina.

Ingredients

- 1 ounce alfalfa leaf

- 1 ounce nettle leaf

- 1 ounce milky oats

- 1 ounce red raspberry leaf

- ½ ounce ashwagandha

- ½ ounce licorice root

Directions

Place all ingredients in a bowl and mix. Store in a mason jar.

To brew a cup of tea: Steep 1 tablespoon of herbs in 1 cup of hot water for 10 minutes, covered.

To brew a large batch: Steep 4 tablespoons of herbs per quart of boiling water for 30 minutes.

Drink 1-4 cups daily.

If you have high blood pressure, omit the licorice.

Gentle Energy Lifting Tea

Gotu kola and licorice support healthy energy, while the other supporting herbs in this tea feed and nourish your tissues, especially the adrenals.

Ingredients

- ½ ounce gotu kola leaf

- ½ ounce nettle leaf

- ½ ounce red raspberry leaf

- ¼ ounce licorice root

- ¼ ounce yellow dock

Directions

Place all ingredients in a bowl and mix. Store in a mason jar.

To brew a cup of tea: Steep 1 tablespoon of herbs in 1 cup of hot water for 10 minutes, covered.

To brew a large batch: Steep 4 tablespoons of herbs per quart of boiling water for 30 minutes.

Drink 1-4 cups daily.

Omega-3 Blueberry Brain Booster

Blueberries are rich with antioxidants, which protect your cells from damage. Avocado and fish oil provide the necessary fat that your brain craves. I like using grass-fed gelatin in my smoothies because it has the benefit of providing protein and the necessary amino acids to help heal damaged tissue.

Ingredients

- 1 cup frozen organic blueberries

- ¼ cup frozen raspberries

- ½ avocado

- ½ banana

- 1-2 teaspoons of fish oil

- 1 teaspoon turmeric powder

- 2 tablespoons grass-fed gelatin

Directions

Place all of your ingredients in a high powered blender and mix until smooth.

Blackberry-Cinnamon Smoothie

Adding to cinnamon to smoothies encourages better blood sugar regulation, which means less crashes in energy. Chia seeds provide brain healthy omega-3 fatty acids and helps keep the bowels regular.

Ingredients

- 1 cup fresh or frozen blackberries

- 1 cup coconut milk or organic whole milk

- 1 teaspoon chia seeds

- ½ teaspoon cinnamon

- 1 handful of spinach

Directions

Place all of your ingredients in a high powered blender and mix until smooth.

Summer Power House Smoothie

I love this smoothie because it is packed with nutrients that supports healing, keeps the bowel regular and tastes amazing!

Ingredients

- 3 organic rainbow chard leaves

- 1 cup organic spinach

- 2 small beets, cooked and peeled

- ¼ cup tart cherries

- ¼ cup blueberries

- 8-10 strawberries

- 4 tablespoons grass-fed gelatin

- ⅛ cup water

Directions

Place your ingredients in the blender with the leaves in first. Process until smooth.

Vanilla Hemp Protein Smoothie

Vanilla naturally elevates the mood and tastes great! The hemp and almond butter give this smoothie a delicious nutty flavor.

Ingredients

- 5 tablespoons hemp seeds

- 2 tablespoons almond butter

- 1 frozen banana

- 1 tablespoon extra-virgin coconut oil

- 1 tablespoon grass-fed gelatin

- 1 teaspoon pure vanilla extract

- 1 pinch of cinnamon

- 1 cup purified water

Directions

Place hempseeds, water, vanilla, coconut oil, almond butter, cinnamon and gelatin in the blender on high and process until the mixture becomes frothy.

Hydrating Smoothie

As a breastfeeding mother I found myself thirsty all the time. I found this smoothie hit the spot, especially on hot days.

Ingredients

- ½ large cucumber, peeled and sliced

- 1 cup frozen cherries

- 1 cup coconut water

- 3 fresh mint leaves

- 2 tablespoons grass-fed gelatin

Directions

Place all of your ingredients in a high powered blender and mix until smooth.

Green Smoothie

Getting enough greens might seem tough in the early weeks postpartum. Whipping up your greens as a beverage is one trick I use when I'm needing a bit more greens.

Ingredients

- 2 cups organic spinach

- 2 romaine lettuce leaves

- ½ avocado

- 1 kiwi, peeled

- ½ green pear

- ¾ cup organic goat kefir, coconut milk or water

- 1 tablespoon fresh squeezed lime juice

Directions

Place your ingredients in the blender with the leaves in first. Process until smooth.

Mono Loco Smoothie

Keep a can of coconut cream in your fridge to make a creamy and delicious morning beverage. When and if you're ready to incorporate regular coffee you can substitute for the decaf.

Ingredients

- 1 banana

- 1 cup chilled coconut cream

- ½ cup cold, decaf coffee

- 2 tablespoons raw cocoa powder

- 1 tablespoon melted, unsalted organic grass-fed butter

Directions

Place all of your ingredients in a high powered blender and mix until smooth.

Pumpkin Pie Smoothie

Pumpkin is an excellent source of vitamin A, which is essential when skin is trying to heal. Vitamin A also supports a healthy immune system.

Ingredients

- ¾ cup pureed pumpkin

- ⅓ cup organic whole milk or coconut milk

- 2 tablespoons fresh ground flax

- ¼ cup coconut water

- 2 teaspoons raw honey

- 2 teaspoons cinnamon

- ½ teaspoon nutmeg

- ½ teaspoon pumpkin pie spice

Directions

Place all of your ingredients in a high powered blender and mix until smooth.

Balsamic Blueberry Gummies

Gelatin is amazing at helping your body heal. These gummies make delicious and quick mommy snacks that provide you with a good dose of protein to quench hunger cravings and sustain your energy.

Ingredients

- ⅔ cup organic balsamic vinegar

- 1 cup fresh organic blueberries

- 4 tablespoons unflavored grass-fed gelatin

Directions

1. Place balsamic vinegar and blueberries into a heavy sauce pan, place on medium heat.

2. Simmer, stirring frequently, until the blueberries are plump.

3. Place the mixture into a high speed blender and blend until smooth.

4. Allow the mixture to cool slightly, mixture should still be warm.

5. Add gelatin and blend until smooth.

6. Pour mixture into a 9x9 glass dish and re-frigerate for an hour. If using candy molds, refrigerate for 30 minutes.

Stress Ease Gummies

The passion flower and lemon balm combined create a calming effect. Pop one or maybe 3 when you are feeling stressed.

Ingredients

- 1 teaspoon passion flower herb

- 1 teaspoon lemon balm herb

- 1 cup water

- ½ cup tart cherry juice

- 2 tablespoons honey

Directions

1. Make a cup of tea with herbs and 1 cup of boiled water. Allow to steep for 10 minutes. Strain and discard the herbs.

2. Combine tea, tart cherry juice, and honey in a small sauce pan over medium-low heat.

3. Slowly add gelatin into the mixture, whisking constantly until all ingredients are well combined.

4. Place silicone candy mold mixture on a cookies sheet for easy transport. Pour mixture into silicone candy mold and place in freezer for 20-30 minutes.

5. Remove gummies from the mold and store in an airtight container.

Prune Chia Seed Pudding

Serves: 1

Eat this as a morning meal or snack on the days your bowels are being a bit stubborn.

Ingredients

- 4-6 prunes

- 1 cup of water

- 2 tablespoons chia seeds

- ¼ teaspoon cinnamon

- ¼ teaspoon nutmeg

Directions

Place prunes and water in a saucepan. Cover and simmer for 15 minutes. Allow to cool and place in a food processor or blender with chia seeds and spices. Puree to your preferred consistency. Enjoy warm or cold.

Blueberry Coconut Yogurt

Serves: 1-2

This is a sneaky way of getting a little more greens into your day. I recommend using curly green kale. The added probiotics also encourage good gut health.

Ingredients

- ½ cup coconut cream, chilled (place in refrigerator overnight)
- Handful of organic blueberries
- 1 large kale leaf, ribs removed
- 1 serving probiotics (powder or capsule, opened)

Directions

Toss everything into a blender or food processor. Blend until the kale pieces are the size you desire. Serve into a bowl and top with berries with extra berries.

Sweet Potato Noodles with Bacon

Serves: 4

Ingredients

- 3-6 slices of bacon

- 2 large sweet potatoes, peeled and spiralized (grated works too!)

- 4 cups of kale, ribs removed and chopped to bite size (smaller for kids)

- ½ onion, diced (optional)

Directions

Chop bacon to desired size and cook in a pan over medium-high heat until it has just almost reached the crispness you desire.

Place your prepped sweet potato in the pan. If you like your sweet potato to have a little crunch, cook for about 5-8 minutes. If you want a softer noodle, cover with a lid, but continue to stir often (so that the sweet potato doesn't stick to the bottom) and cook for about 10 minutes. Take a nibble from the noodles while you are cooking to find which level of cooking you desire.

Add kale, stirring often and cook for another 2-3 minutes.

Serve hot and enjoy.

Plantain Pancakes

Serves: 4

I really enjoy a fresh nut butter and a dollop of apple sauce on top of my pancakes instead of syrup.

Ingredients

- 2 large green plantains, pureed
- 4 eggs
- 3 tablespoons coconut oil (and extra to cook pancakes)
- ⅛ teaspoons salt
- ½ teaspoons baking soda
- 1 teaspoon cinnamon
- ½ teaspoon nutmeg
- 2 teaspoons vanilla

Directions

Place peeled plantains in food processor or blender. Add eggs and blend until smooth, batter-like consistency.

Add the remaining ingredients and blend on high for an additional 2 minutes.

Place 1 tablespoon coconut oil in a pan, heat on medium-high. Once the oil is warmed, add batter to the size of pancake you wish to have.

Cook 4-5 minutes then flip and cook another 1-2 minutes.

Fruit and Nut Breakfast Cookies

Don't let the name fool you—you can eat these anytime! I kept these in my fridge for whenever the breastfeeding hunger crept up.

Ingredients

- 2 large ripe plantains
- ½ cup unsweetened applesauce
- 2 tablespoons ghee
- 4 pitted dates
- ⅓ cup coconut flour
- 1 teaspoon baking soda
- 1 ½ teaspoons lemon juice
- ½ cup finely shredded dried coconut
- 3 tablespoons dried apricots, chopped
- 3 tablespoons raisins
- ¼ cup walnut pieces
- 2 teaspoon cinnamon
- 1 teaspoon vanilla

Directions

1. Preheat oven to 350 degrees F. In a food processor, puree the plantains, dates, applesauce, and ghee until smooth.

2. Add coconut flour, baking soda, lemon juice, cinnamon, vanilla. Pulse the food processor 6 times to combine.

3. Add the raisins, apricot, walnuts and shredded coconut. Pulse the food processor once, maybe twice to combine, but don't over due it or the fruit will become a mash.

4. Using a large spoon, scoop dough onto a cookie sheet lined with parchment. Shape cookies using your hands. These cookies do not spread with baking.

5. Bake for 18-20 minutes. Let the cookies cool completely. Store in an airtight container in the fridge for one week.

Mallory's Simple Bone Broth Recipe

Makes: About 4 quarts

Ingredients

- 5 lb. bones (see below)

- 1 medium, white onion

- 2 medium carrots, chopped

- 3-4 stalks celery

- 1 leek, halved

- 7 garlic cloves, smashed

- 2 tablespoons apple cider vinegar

- 1 teaspoon cracked whole black peppercorns

- 6 sprigs parsley

- 6 sprigs thyme

- 2 bay leaves

- 1 teaspoon turmeric powder

- Salt to taste

A note on bones

You can use beef, veal, lamb, bison, buffalo, pork, goose, turkey, chicken, or fish (including the head) bones to make bone broth, according to your taste. For meat bones, get a variety, asking your local butcher for marrow bones, oxtail, and "soup bones." However, I highly recommend starting with fowl, as it tends to produce the mildest flavor. Save the bones from a whole chicken or turkey (after you've eaten the meat) and add a few chicken feet and necks for extra collagen and nutrients. Always source the highest quality bones from pastured and/or grass-fed animals.

Directions

1. Cut onion, carrots, celery and leek into chunks and add to a crockpot with the bones.

2. Add smashed garlic and apple cider vinegar.

3. Fill the crockpot to the brim with filtered water.

4. Cook broth anywhere from 24-48 hours on "low" in the crockpot (If working on a stovetop, you'll want to keep it on a very low simmer, covered, for the same amount

of time. If you don't feel comfortable leaving the stove on at night, turn it to the very lowest setting, then turn it back up in the morning.)

5. When you have about 2 hours left, add herbs/spices and make sure they're covered with liquid.

6. After the allotted time, turn the heat off and let the broth cool down until it's safe to handle.

7. Strain the liquid into a large bowl and discard all solids. From here, you can transfer your broth into smaller containers and fridge or freeze. Keep bone broth for up to one week in the fridge or freeze for up to six months.

Medicinal Mushroom Soup

Serves: 4

This soup is incredibly powerful for building your immune system and providing necessary nutrients to support your overall health.

Ingredients

- 1 large reishi mushroom

- 1 tablespoon fresh grated ginger

- 3 garlic cloves, minced

- 1 medium yellow onion, chopped

- 1 pound shitake mushrooms, chopped

- 6 carrots, chopped

- 4 stocks of celery

- 3 boneless chicken thighs

- 1 boneless chicken breast

- 8 cups bone broth

- Salt and pepper to taste

Directions

1. Place chicken in the pot with bone broth, bring to a boil over a medium high heat. Reduce heat and simmer for 20 minutes. Remove chicken and set aside.

2. Place reishi mushroom in the pot and simmer for 20 minutes covered. Using a slotted spoon, remove reishi mushroom. (Note: If you don't have time for this step you can skip the reishi.) While reishi mushroom is simmering, shred chicken.

3. Add the rest of the ingredients and simmer for 10-20 minutes.

4. Add chicken back to the pot and serve.

Beef Heart Meatballs

Serves: 4

Beef heart is an excellent source of iron, CoQ10 and B vitamins. This recipe combines the heart with ground beef making it undetectable and highly palatable.

Ingredients

- 1 pound grass-fed ground beef

- ½ pound grass-fed ground beef heart

- 3 large eggs, beaten

- 1 large onion, diced

- 2 garlic cloves, minced

- 1 teaspoon Pink Himalayan salt

- 1 teaspoon black pepper

- 1 teaspoon dried parsley

- 1 teaspoon dried thyme

Directions

1. Preheat oven to 350 F

2. Place beef in a large bowl. Add all ingredients and mix well with your hands.

3. Form into small, meatball shape.

4. Place on a cookie sheet in the oven. Bake 15 minutes.

Slow Cooker Beef & Chicken Liver Chili

Serves: 4

Liver helps replenish iron stores, provide ample vitamin A and vitamin B6. The combination of flavors in this recipe create a compliment to the subtle flavor of the liver.

Ingredients

- 2 pounds grass-fed ground beef

- ½ pound ground pastured chicken livers

- 2 onions, diced

- 4 garlic cloves, minced

- 3 cans (14.5 oz) diced tomatoes

- 1 can (6 oz) tomato paste

- 2 zucchini, diced

- 1 cup carrots, finely diced

- 1 orange bell pepper, diced

- 1 ½ cups water or bone broth

- 2 tablespoons paprika

- 1 tablespoon chili powder

- 1 tablespoon cumin

- 1 tablespoon dried oregano

- 1 tablespoon dried basil

- 1 teaspoon black pepper

Directions

Combine ingredients into a 6 quart crockpot. Cook on a low setting for 8 hours. You can stir twice during this time. Salt to taste.

30 Minute Curry

This recipes combines medicinal seasoning that reduces inflammation, support breast milk production and digestive upset.

Ingredients

For the Curry:

- 1 pound uncooked prawns

- 1 tablespoon coconut

- 1 small onion

- 4 cloves garlic

- 1 tablespoon fresh grated ginger

- ½ cup broccoli florets

- ½ cup diced carrots

- ¼ cup diced tomato

- ½ cup snow peas

- 1 teaspoon dried coriander

- 1 ½ teaspoons cumin

- ⅛ teaspoon ground nutmeg

- ¾ teaspoon turmeric powder

- ¼ teaspoon fennel seed

- 3 tablespoons fish sauce

- 1 can full fat coconut milk

- 1 cup bone broth or chicken stock

- Sea salt and black pepper to taste

Directions

1. Place ginger, garlic, onion (chop into pieces), spices, fish sauce and ginger into the food processor until a paste forms.

2. Add paste bone broth, coconut milk, and coconut oil. Stir while bringing to a simmer then reduce heat slightly to medium-low. Add broccoli, carrots, and prawns Cook for 8 minutes.

3. Add the snow peas and tomatoes. Cook another 4-5 minutes. Prawns will turn a light pink and be firm to the touch.

4. Salt and pepper as needed.

5. Serve over white rice.

Zucchini and Sweet Potato Frittata

Serves: 4

Frittatas were one of my go to dishes when I had my son. They are easy to create and made for a quick all in one meal.

Ingredients

- 2 tablespoons cultured ghee or coconut oil

- 8 pastured eggs

- 1 large sweet potato, peeled and cut into slices

- 1 red bell pepper, diced

- 2 zucchinis, sliced

- 2 tablespoons fresh parsley

- Salt and pepper to taste

Directions

1. Heat oil over medium-low heat. Add sweet potato slices and cook until soft, about 7-10 minutes.

2. Add bell pepper and zucchini and cook for another 3 minutes.

3. While the potatoes are cooking, whisk eggs in a bowl. Season eggs with salt and pepper.

4. Pour eggs over your vegetables and cook on low heat until eggs are cooked through, about 10 minutes.

5. Cut the frittata into wedges and top with fresh parsley.

APPENDIX B: DAILY NUTRIENT REQUIREMENTS FOR LACTATION VS. PREGNANCY

B Vitamins

Nutrient	Lactation	Pregnancy	Sources
Thiamin (B1)	1.4 mg	1.4 mg	Blackstrap molasses, spinach, cauliflower, most nuts, sunflower seeds, peas, avocado, pork
Riboflavin (B2)	1.6 mg	1.4 mg	Spinach, beet greens, eggs, almonds
Niacin (B3)	17 mg	18 mg	Turkey, chicken, salmon, sardines, organ meats
Pantothenic acid (B5)	7 mg	6 mg	Shiitake mushrooms, avocado, sweet potatoes, chicken
Pyridoxane (B6)	2.0 mg	1.9 mg	Liver and other organ meats, fish, poultry, egg yolk, walnuts, banana, prunes, potatoes, cauliflower, cabbage, avocado
Biotin (B7)	35 mcg	30 mcg	Egg yolk, liver, kidney, almonds, walnuts
Folate (B9)	500 mcg	800 mcg	Asparagus, spinach, broccoli, lentils
Cyanocobalimin (B12)	2.8 mcg	2.6 mcg	Organ meats, trout, herring, mackerel, crab, oysters, egg yolk, grass-fed yogurt

Vitamin C

Nutrient	Lactation	Pregnancy	Sources
Vitamin C	120 mg	85 mg	Citrus, kiwi, strawberries, tomato, sweet red pepper, broccoli, potato, spinach

Fat Soluble Vitamins

Nutrient	Lactation	Pregnancy	Sources
Vitamin A	4,333 IU	2,567 IU	Liver, fish liver oil, egg yolks, raw & grass-fed whole milk, cream, butter
Vitamin D`	600 IU	600 IU	Sunlight, pink salmon, mackerel, sardines, egg yolk, butter
Vitamin E	28.5 IU	22.5 IU	Olive oil, almonds, hazelnuts, spinach, carrots, avocado
Vitamin K	90 mcg	90 mcg	Kale, Swiss chard, parsley, broccoli, spinach, watercress, green-leafed lettuce

Major Minerals

Nutrient	Lactation	Pregnancy	Sources
Calcium	1,000 mg	1,000 mg	Sardines, Chinese cabbage, figs, orange, kale, broccoli
Magnesium	320 mg	360 mg	Mackeral, spinach, almonds, Swiss chard, hazelnuts, banana
Phosphorous	700 mg	700 mg	Salmon, halibut, turkey, chicken, beef, almonds, egg
Potassium	5,100 mg	4,700 mg	Banana, potato, prunes, orange, tomato, artichoke, acorn squash, spinach, sunflower seeds, almonds
Sodium	1,500 mg	1,500 mg	Seafood, beef, poultry, celery, beets, carrots, artichokes, kelp and other sea vegetables.

Trace Minerals

Nutrient	Lactation	Pregnancy	Sources
Chromium	45 mcg	30 mcg	Broccoli, green beans, potatoes, beef, turkey
Copper	1.3 mg	1 mg	Beef liver, oysters, crab, clams, cashews, sunflower seeds, hazelnuts, almonds, mushrooms
Fluoride	3 mg	3 mg	Black tea, crab (canned), fish, chicken
Iodine	290 mcg	220 mcg	Iodized salt, cod, shrimp, tuna, egg, turkey, seaweed
Iron	9 mg	27 mg	Meat, poultry, fish
Manganese	2.6 mg	2 mg	Pineapple, pecans, almonds, spinach, sweet potato, green tea, black tea
Molybdenum	50 mcg	50 mcg	Peas, most nuts, lentils
Selenium	70 mcg	60 mcg	Brazil nuts, tuna, oysters, clams, halibut, shrimp, salmon, pork, beef, chicken, sunflower seeds
Zinc	12 mg	11 mg	Oysters, beef, crab, pork, turkey, chicken, cashews, almonds

Other Nutrients

Nutrient	Lactation	Pregnancy	Sources
Choline	550 mg	450 mg	Beef liver, beef, egg, scallop, salmon, chicken, cod, shrimp, Brussels sprouts, broccoli
Fiber	29 g	28 g	Lentils, artichokes, prunes, almonds
Omega-3 Fatty Acids	1.3 g	1.4 g	Herring, salmon, sardines, salmon

Source: Linus Pauling Institute

APPENDIX C: RESOURCES

Visit Dr. Jolene Brighten's website for supplement recommendations, free downloads, online programs, and more!

www.drbrighten.com

To learn how you can work with Dr. Brighten, please contact info@drbrighten.com

Birth Options

Birth Network National
www.birthnetwork.org

Childbirth Connection
www.childbirthconnection.org

Choices in Childbirth
www.choicesinchildbirth.org

Coalition for Improving Maternity Services
www.motherfriendly.org

Doulas of North America International
www.dona.org

Happy Healthy Child
www.happyhealthychild.com

Cesarean Section

Belly Bandit
www.bellybandit.com

Childbirth Connection
www.childbirthconnection.org

C-Section Recovery
www.csectionrecovery.com

International Cesarean Awareness Network
www.ican-online.org

Vaginal Birth After Cesarean (V-BAC)
www.vbac.com

Childbirth Education

Birthing From Within
www.birthingfromwithin.com

The Bradley Method
www.bradleybirth.com

Choices in Birth
www.choicesinchildbirth.org

Hypnobirthing
www.hypnobirthing.com

Lamaze International
www.lamaze.org

Breast Feeding Support

Ameda
www.ameda.com

Human Milk for Human Babies
www.hm4hb.net

Kelly Mom
www.kellymom.com

La Leche League International
www.lalecheleague.org

Milkin' Mamas
www.milknmamas.com

U.S. Department of Health
www.womenshealth.gov

Nutrition & Recipes

Against All Grain by Danielle Walker

Deliciously Organic by Carrie Vitt

The Paleo Approach by Sarah Ballantyne

Nom Nom Paleo by Michelle Tam

One-Pot Paleo by Jenny Castaneda

Juli Bauer's Paleo Cookbook by Juli Bauer

Make it Paleo II by Hayley Mason

The Performance Paleo Cookbook by Stephanie Gaudreau

The Kitchn Cookbook by Sara Kate Gillingham

The Ancestral Table by Russ Crandall

The Zen Belly Cookbook by Simone Miller

It Starts With Food by Dallas Hartwig & Melissa Hartwig

Practical Paleo by Diane Sanfilippo

Nourishing Traditions by Sally Fallon

Herbal Products

Earth Mama Angel Baby
www.earthmamaangelbaby.com

Gaia Herbs
www.gaiaherbs.com

Herb Pharm
www.herb-pharm.com

Mountain Rose Herbs
www.mountainroseherbs.com

Wish Garden Herbs
www.wishgardenherbs.com

Wise Woman Herbals
www.wisewomanherbals.com

Postpartum Support

Center for Women's Mental Health
www.womensmentalhealth.org

Beyond Meds
www.beyondmeds.com

Integrative Medicine for Mental Health
www.integrativemedicineformentalhealth.com

Postpartum Support International
www.postpartum.net Helpline: 1-800-944-4PPD (4773)

Recovery, Inc
www.recoveryinternational.org Helpline: 1-312-337-5661

Women's Mental Health Center
www.womensmentalhealth.org

Pelvic Floor & Exercise Support

Katy Bowman
www.katysays.com

Leslie Howard, RYT
www.lesliehowardyoga.com

Tami Lynn Kent, MPT, Creator of Holistic Pelvic Care™
www.wildfeminine.com

The Dia Method
www.thediamethod.com

Practitioner Referrals

American Association of Naturopathic Physicians
www.naturopathic.org

Gastroenterology Association of Naturopathic Physicians
www.gastroanp.org

Holistic Pediatric Association
www.hpadirectory.org

Institute for Functional Medicine
www.functionalmedicine.org

Integrative Medicine for Mental Health
www.integrativemedicineformentalhealth.com

Pediatric Association of Naturopathic Physicians
www.pedanp.org

Primal Docs
www.primaldocs.com

Thyroid Change
www.thyroidchange.org

Parenting Support

Dream Team Baby
www.dreamteambaby.com

Healthy Child
www.healthychild.org

Holistic Moms Network
www.holisticmoms.org

Kelly Mom
www.kellymom.com

National Vaccine Information Center
www.nvic.org

Pathways to Family Wellness
www.pathwaystofamilywellness.org

Seedlings Group
www.seedlingsgroup.com

Citations

[1] McCoy, Bonnie A., Roberta E. Bleiler, and Margaret A. Ohlson. "Iron Content of Intact Placentas and Cords." The American Journal of Clinical Nutrition 9, no. 5 (1961): 613-15.

[2] Abbott, P., A.c. Thompson, E.j. Ferguson, J.c. Doerr, J.a. Tarapacki, P.j. Kostyniak, J.a. Syracuse, D.m. Cartonia, and M.b. Kristal. "Placental Opioid-enhancing Factor (POEF): Generalizability of Effects." Physiology & Behavior: 933-40.

[3] Dipirro, Jean M, and Mark B Kristal. "Placenta Ingestion by Rats Enhances δ- and ϰ-opioid Antinociception, but Suppresses μ-opioid Antinociception." Brain Research: 22-33.

[4] Selander, Jodi, Allison Cantor, Sharon M. Young, and Daniel C. Benyshek. "Human Maternal Placentophagy: A Survey of Self-Reported Motivations and Experiences Associated with Placenta Consumption." Ecology of Food and Nutrition: 93-115.

ACKNOWLEDGEMENTS

For me, writing a book as mother with a very busy practice wouldn't be possible with out ample support. Thank you so much to my husband, Bryce for supporting me through many late nights, tireless weekends and for always being willing to read and re-read everything I write.

Thank you to Mallory Leone for being an excellent side kick and helping the book become a reality.

Thank you to my most wonderful in-law, Warren and Kathy Hamrick who have always supported me and have been such wonderful grandparents. A special thank you to Kathy for refilling my birth tub with hot water and feeding all my birth attendants.

Thank you Liliana Barzola-Reed for being my

energetic mentor and holding space for me through life's challenges.

Thank you Tami Lynn Kent for teaching me the art, the medicine and the practice of Holistic Pelvic Care™. And I thank you for being my pelvic care provider following the birth of my son.

I'd also like to acknowledge some of my mentors who have taught me so much and always believed in my abilities: Dr. Dick Thom, Dr. Kimberly Windstar, and Dr. Amy Bader.

Special big thanks to Dr. Jenny Maurer, Dr. Amanda Roe, Dr. Megan Golani, and Dr. Brook Schales for being my guides as I brought my son into this world.